AIDS Dx/Rx

NOTICE

Treament for selected infections

Organism	Treatment	Dose	Duration or comments
Candida species			
Oral	Clotrimazole troche *or* Nystatin *or* Ketoconazole	10-mg troche 4 to 6 times per day 500,000 units 4 to 6 times per day 200–400 mg per day	Until clinically resolved; then taper to maintenance therapy
Esophageal	Ketoconazole *or* Amphotericin B	400 mg per day 0.3 mg/kg per day	Until clinically resolved; use amphotericin B if disease is severe or if no response to oral therapy is obtained; maintenance therapy needed
Cryptococcus neoformans			
Meningitis	Amphotericin B*	0.4–0.6 mg/kg per day *or* 0.8–1.0 mg/kg every other day	For 6 weeks or total dose of 1.5–2.0 g followed by lifelong maintenance therapy; optimal dose for maintenance unknown; consider amphotericin B, 100 mg/week, or fluconazole, 100 mg/day
Mycobacterium avium intracellulare	No known effective treatment		
M. tuberculosis	Isoniazid Rifampin Pyrazinamide (PZA)	5 mg/kg per day 9 mg/kg per day 25 mg/kg per day	Use three drugs for 2 months, then discontinue PZA; continue two drugs for a minimum of 9 months
Toxoplasma gondii	Pyrimethamine *and* Sulfadiazine *and* Folinic acid	50–100 mg loading dose; then 25–50 mg per day 4 g per day 5 mg per day	For 3–6 months followed by lifelong maintenance therapy; optimal maintenance dose unknown
Herp[illegible]lex vir[illegible]	Acyclovir		
Tre[illegible]ent		400 mg every 8 h PO *or* 5 mg/kg every 8 h IV	
Prophylaxis		200–400 mg every 8 h PO	
Varicella-zoster virus	Acyclovir	10 mg/kg every 8 h IV	
CMV	Ganciclovir	5 mg/kg every 12 h; then 5 mg/kg per day IV‡	

Note: Some regimens are not approved by the FDA for the treatment of viral infections.

*Or fluconazole; see text.

†Genital or mucocutaneous presentations.

‡14-day induction regimen followed by daily maintenance.

AIDS Dx/Rx

Editors

King K. Holmes, Ph.D.
Director, Center for AIDS and Sexually Transmitted Diseases
Professor of Medicine, Adjunct Professor of
Epidemiology and Microbiology
University of Washington

Lawrence Corey, M.D.
Head, Division of Virology
Professor, Departments of Laboratory Medicine,
Microbiology, Medicine, Pediatrics
University of Washington

Ann C. Collier, M.D.
Medical Director, AIDS Clinic, Harborview Medical Center
Assistant Professor of Medicine, University of Washington

H. Hunter Handsfield, M.D.
Director, Sexually Transmitted Disease Control Program
Seattle-King County Department of Public Health
Professor of Medicine, Adjunct Professor of Epidemiology
University of Washington

Associate Editor

Donna Z. Mirkes, M.S.
University of Washington

McGRAW-HILL
Health Professions Division

New York St. Louis San Francisco Colorado Springs Auckland Bogotá
Caracas Hamburg Lisbon London Madrid Mexico Milan Montreal
New Delhi Paris San Juan São Paulo Singapore Sydney Tokyo Toronto

AIDS Dx/Rx

1 2 3 4 5 6 7 8 9 0 DOC DOC 9 8 7 6 5 4 3 2 1 0

ISBN 0-07-029678-2

This book was set in Times Roman by Kachina Typesetting Inc.
The editors were William Day and Mariapaz Ramos-Englis;
the production supervisor was Robert R. Laffler.
The text and cover were designed and the project was supervised by M 'N O Production Services, Inc.
R. R. Donnelley and Sons was printer and binder.

The material contained in this book represents an extension of material presented in two earlier editions of *AIDS: A Guide for the Primary Physician*. The first edition was published as Volume 13, Number 1 (Winter 1987) of *University of Washington Medicine*, published by the University of Washington School of Medicine, Seattle, Arno G. Motulsky, editor. A revised version was subsequently published in 1988 by the University of Washington Press, Seattle, King K. Holmes and Arno G. Motulsky, editors.

Permission to reprint material from the 1988 version has generously been granted by the University of Washington Press.

Photographs provided by: All of You Photographic Services (p. 186); Doug Arditti (p. 212); UW Department of Medicial History and Ethics (p. 218); James L. Kinyoun (p. 120); Mary Levin (p. 215); Cynthia Taylor (p. 210).

Library of Congress Cataloging-in-Publication Data

AIDS Dx/Rx / edited by King K. Holmes . . . [et al.].
p. cm.
ISBN 0-07 029678-2
1. AIDS (Disease) I. Holmes, King K.
RC607.A26A345734 1990
616.97'92—dc20 89-13888
CIP

Contents

Contributors

Heather Andersen, R.N., M.N.
Lecturer, University of Washington School of Social Work and School of Nursing; and Staff Member, University of Washington AIDS Education and Training Center

Fredrick H. Bahls, M.D., Ph.D.
Acting Assistant Professor, Division of Neurology and Department of Physiology and Biophysics, University of Washington; and Attending Neurologist, Seattle Veterans Administration Medical Center

William B. Bateman, Jr., M.D.
Director, Social Internal Medicine Residency and Assistant Professor, Departments of Medicine, Epidemiology, and Social Medicine, Montefiore Medical Center—Albert Einstein College of Medicine

Sandra Burchett, M.D., M.S.
Acting Instructor, Department of Pediatrics, University of Washington

Connie Celum, M.D., M.P.H.
Senior Fellow, Infectious Diseases Division, Department of Medicine, University of Washington

Ann C. Collier, M.D.
Assistant Professor, Department of Medicine, University of Washington; and Medical Director, AIDS Clinic, Harborview Medical Center

Robert W. Coombs, M.D., Ph.D.
Acting Assistant Professor, Department of Laboratory Medicine, University of Washington

Lawrence Corey, M.D.
Head, Division of Virology and Professor, Departments of Laboratory Medicine, Microbiology, Medicine, and Pediatrics, University of Washington

Terence C. Gayle, M.D.
Clinical Assistant Professor, Department of Psychiatry and Behavioral Sciences, University of Washington; Psychiatric Consultant, Harborview Medical Center Infectious Disease Clinic; Staff Member, University of Washington AIDS Education and Training Center; and in private practice, Seattle

Lewayne D. Gilchrist, Ph.D.
Associate Dean of Research and Associate Professor, University of Washington School of Social Work; and Staff Member, University of Washington AIDS Education and Training Center

Lynn Goldstein, M.D.
Resident, Department of Pathology, University of Washington

H. Hunter Handsfield, M.D.
Director, Sexually Transmitted Disease Control Program, Seattle-King County Department of Public Health; and Professor, Department of Medicine and Adjunct Professor, Department of Epidemiology, University of Washington

Frederick M. Hecht, M.D.
Instructor, Division of Infectious Disease, Department of Medicine, AIDS Center, Montefiore Medical Center–Albert Einstein College of Medicine

King K. Holmes, M.D., Ph.D.
Director, Center for AIDS and Sexually Transmitted Diseases; Professor, Department of Medicine and Adjunct Professor, Departments of Epidemiology and Microbiology, University of Washington

Harold W. Jaffe, M.D.
Deputy Director for Science, AIDS Program, Center for Infectious Diseases, Centers for Disease Control

John Jewett, M.D.
Internist, currently attending the Harvard School of Public Health Master's in Public Health Program

Albert R. Jonsen, Ph.D.
Professor of Ethics in Medicine, and Chairman, Department of Medical History and Ethics, University of Washington

Michael G. Katze, Ph.D.
Core Staff Scientist, University of Washington Regional Primate Research Center; and Assistant Professor, Department of Microbiology, University of Washington

Ann M. Kimball, M.D., M.P.H.
Regional Advisor on AIDS, Pan American Health Organization

Joan Kreiss, M.D., M.S.P.H.
Assistant Professor, Departments of Medicine and of Epidemiology, University of Washington

Patricia Lynch, R.N., M.B.A.
Infection Control Practioner, Harborview Medical Center; and Adjunct Clinical Instructor, Department of Epidemiology, University of Washington

John Mills, M.D.
Professor, Department of Medicine, University of California, San Francisco; and Chief of Infectious Diseases, San Francisco General Hospital

Joseph F. O'Neill, M.D., M.P.H.
Chief Medical Officer, Division of HIV Services of the Health Resources and Services Administration; and Former Chief Resident, Primary Care Internal Medicine Program, University of Washington

J. Brian O'Toole, Ph.D.
Director, Continuing Medical Education, University of Washington

Paul G. Ramsey, M.D.
Associate Chairman and Associate Professor, Department of Medicine; and Continuing Medical Education Advisory Committee, University of Washington

Julia R. Smith, M.D.
Internist in private practice, Seattle; and Clinical Assistant Professor, Department of Medicine, University of Washington

Walter E. Stamm, M.D.
Head, Infectious Diseases Division; and Acting Head, Department of Medicine, Harborview Medical Center; and Professor, Department of Medicine and Adjunct Professor, Department of Epidemiology, University of Washington

Teresa A. Tartaglione, Pharm.D.
Assistant Professor, Department of Pharmacy Practice, University of Washington

Heather Watts, M.D.
Assistant Professor, Department of Obstetrics and Gynecology, University of Washington

Robert W. Wood, M.D.
Director, AIDS Control Programs, Seattle-King County Department of Public Health; and Associate Professor, Department of Medicine, University of Washington

Preface

This small handbook began life as a primer for primary clinicians, first published in 1988 by the University of Washington's medical journal, *UW Medicine,* and then reprinted under the title *AIDS: A Guide for The Primary Care Physicians* by the University of Washington Press. Distributed to approximately 25,000 clinicians in the Northwest, it was well received and reviewed and seemed to fill a distinct need not yet met by other books on AIDS.

We therefore decided to update the book in the fall of 1989 as a set of practical patient-management guidelines in an easily accessible format. Several new chapters were added to deal with common clinical problems, such as testing and counseling; management of the asymptomatic, HIV-seropositive patient; management of common opportunistic infections; and management of perinatal and pediatric HIV infection. The book is intended for primary clinicians who manage patients with HIV infection in a variety of hospital or ambulatory settings. Because management of HIV infection and AIDS is changing so quickly, brief discussions of practical options and the theoretical framework for possible future directions have been necessary. References are provided, not to support the necessarily arbitrary recommendations given, but to provide access to more detailed information on important topics.

The first few chapters provide background information on the global and national epidemiology and the virology of HIV infection, necessary for understanding subsequent chapters on clinical aspects of patient management. We have attempted to orient these early chapters to the clinician. Thus, for example, Chapter 1 focuses on the prevalence of and risk factors for HIV infection in developing countries, when to suspect HIV-2 infection, differences in the clinical manifestations of HIV infection in developing and developed countries, and advice for travelers concerned about the risk of HIV infection.

The remaining chapters deal directly with management of various common aspects of HIV infection, including prevention of nosocomial transmission of HIV. Final sections provide 9 hours of CME credit through the University of Washington and list further useful resources for clinicians who deal with HIV infection and need access to further consultation in this rapidly changing field.

We particularly thank Dr. Arno G. Motulsky, who provided the stimulus to develop the handbook, who participated in editing the edition published by the University of Washington Press, and who, coincidentally, appears to have collected the earliest serum specimen known to contain serum antibody to HIV in Zaire in 1959. We also thank David W. Johnson, Laurie W. Johnson, and Andrew D. Blair for their assistance.

King K. Holmes
Seattle, Washington
November 1989

1

Epidemiology of AIDS and HIV Infection in the United States

H. Hunter Handsfield
Harold W. Jaffe

Before the cause of acquired immunodeficiency syndrome (AIDS) was identified, a definition of AIDS was developed by the Centers for Disease Control (CDC) for the purpose of epidemiologic surveillance. In essence, AIDS was defined by the occurrence of certain serious systemic infections or malignancies predictive of a defect in cell-mediated immunity in a person without a known cause for immune deficiency. Subsequent modifications added a requirement for documentation of infection with human immunodeficiency virus (HIV), permitted presumptive diagnoses of some opportunistic infections, and added certain manifestations to the case definition. It was originally assumed and subsequently confirmed that overt AIDS, according to this definition, encompasses a minority of all HIV infections, although it now appears likely that most persons with HIV infection eventually progress to overtly symptomatic disease. This chapter reviews the epidemiology of AIDS and HIV infection in the United States. The global epidemiology of HIV infection is described in Chap. 2.

REPORTED AIDS CASES AND PROJECTIONS

Through November 1989, 115,158 cases of AIDS in the United States had been reported to the CDC. Of these, 68,441 persons (59.4 percent) were known to have died, including 87 percent of those diagnosed before 1986. Pediatric patients (< 13 years old) accounted for 1947 cases (1.7 percent of the total) and 1059 of the deaths. Table 1-1 displays the incidence of AIDS from December 1988 through November 1989 in the 20 metropolitan areas

Table 1-1. Reported AIDS cases in the 20 United States metropolitan areas with the highest incidences from December 1988 through November 1989

Metropolitan area	Incidence rate* December 1988–November 1989	Cumulative cases through November 1989
San Francisco, CA	107.9	7,224
San Juan, PR	73.9	1,903
New York, NY	63.7	22,573
Jersey City, NJ	61.5	1,376
Newark, NJ	52.3	3,339
Miami, FL	47.9	2,893
Fort Lauderdale, FL	47.4	1,547
West Palm Beach, FL	39.9	1,024
Atlanta, GA	33.3	2,231
Los Angeles, CA	26.4	8,079
Houston, TX	26.4	3,284
Washington, DC	22.8	3,158
Austin, TX	22.8	456
New Orleans, LA	22.1	1,003
Dallas, TX	20.8	1,847
Middlesex, NJ	20.8	635
San Diego, CA	20.5	1,584
Seattle, WA	20.1	1,149
Monmouth–Ocean City, NJ	19.2	465
Baltimore, MD	19.1	1,141
Total (U.S.)	14.2	115,158

*Reported cases per 100,000 population.

with the highest incidence of the disease during this interval and the cumulative number of cases in each area. Figure 1-1 shows the incidence of reported AIDS from August 1988 through July 1988 for the 50 states, Puerto Rico, and the District of Columbia.

The rate of reported new AIDS cases accelerated through 1984, followed by continuing but less sharp increases through late-1989. This trend is believed to be partly due to a declining rate of new cases among homosexually active men.[1, 2] There may also be reduced reporting of cases as more cases are diagnosed outside the hospital setting and as the epidemic stretches available health care resources. In addition, the increasing use of prophylactic antimicrobial therapy to prevent opportunistic infections has probably prevented or delayed some cases of HIV infection in their progression to overt AIDS.

Computer modeling, based on the cases reported through June 1987, projects a total of 365,000 cases through 1992 (Fig. 1-2), with 263,000 cumulative deaths.[3] An estimated 80,000 new cases and 66,000 deaths will

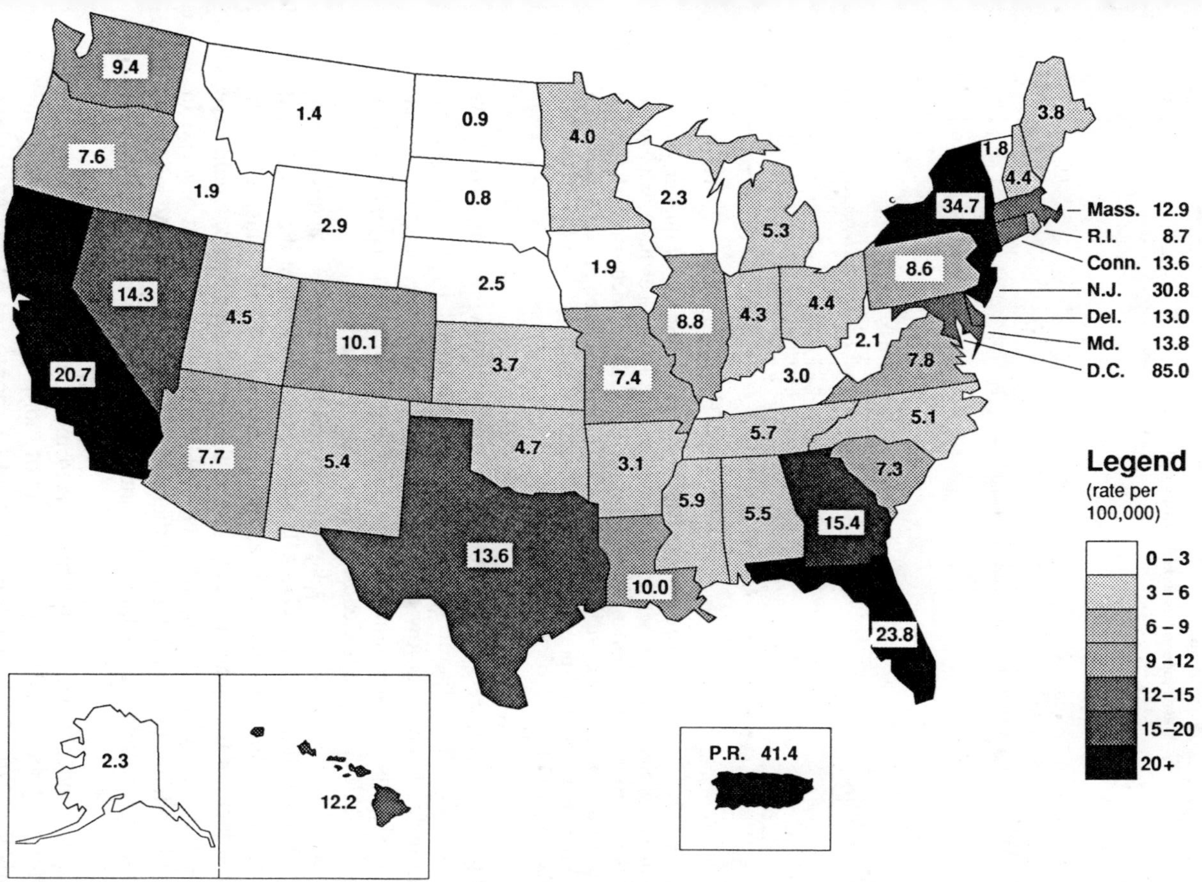

Figure 1-1. AIDS annual incidence rates per 100,000 population for cases reported to the CDC, August 1988 through July 1989. (Source: Centers for Disease Control HIV/AIDS Surveillance Report, August 1989.)

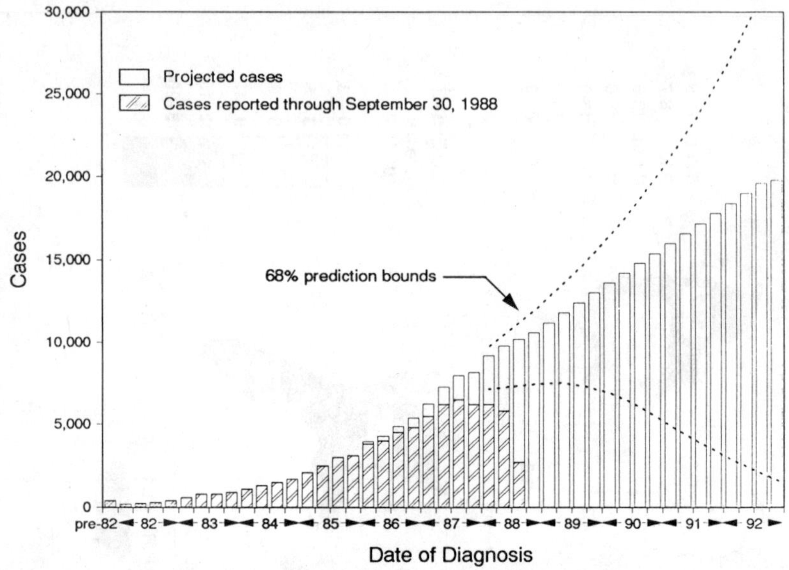

Figure 1-2. Incidence of reported AIDS in the United States by quarter year of diagnosis, projected from cases reported through June 1987 (open bars), with actual incidence from cases reported through September 1988 (shaded bars). (Reprinted with permission from Karon JM, Dondero TJ, Curran JW. The projected incidence of AIDS and estimated prevalence of HIV infection in the United States. *J AIDS* 1988;1:542–550.)

occur during 1992, and 102,000 persons will be living with AIDS. As shown, the precision of these projections, reflected by the 68 percent confidence bounds, is low beyond 2 years. In addition, it is possible that increasing use of zidovudine in early HIV infection may delay progression to overt AIDS and significantly affect these projections.

Because there is usually a lapse of several years between acquisition of HIV and development of overt AIDS (see Chap. 8), most of these projected cases will occur in persons already infected with HIV. Thus, complete curtailment of transmission at this time, if it could be achieved, would have only a modest effect on the number of AIDS cases in the next 5 years. In addition, these estimates ignore other clinically significant HIV infections requiring medical care which substantially outnumber the cases of overt AIDS.

The standard measure of age-adjusted mortality, designed to gauge the differential social and economic impact of mortality in young people, is the statistic "years of potential life lost" (YPLL) prior to age 65. For example, a death at age 40 is weighted more heavily than one at age 60, and deaths after age 65 do not contribute to YPLL calculations. Although the contributions of most diseases (e.g., cardiac disease, trauma) to YPLL fluctuate modestly over time, that due to AIDS has climbed rapidly since the epidemic was recognized. In 1986 AIDS was the eighth leading overall cause of YPLL in the United States and the seventh leading cause in men. By 1992 AIDS will be the second leading cause of YPLL overall and the first or second leading cause in men, roughly equaling the YPLL due to accidents and trauma.[1, 2]

AGE, GENDER, AND RACIAL AND ETHNIC CHARACTERISTICS OF PATIENTS WITH AIDS

Among adults, the age distribution, the ratio of men to women with AIDS, and the distribution of cases according to race and ethnic background are indirect reflections of the modes of transmission of HIV and of differences in the frequency of risk behaviors in various populations. Almost 90 percent of reported AIDS cases in the United States have occurred in persons 20–49 years old at the time of diagnosis; the modal age group, accounting for 24.6 percent of all reported cases, is 30–34.[1, 2] Ninety-one percent of cases have occurred in men. Table 1-2 shows the distribution of reported cases according to race and ethnicity through November 1989. The risk of AIDS is substantially higher for blacks and Hispanics than for whites; together these groups make up less than 20 percent of the U.S. population, but they account for 42 percent of reported AIDS cases.

RISK GROUPS

Table 1-3 shows the hierarchical HIV exposure categories of adults with AIDS in the United States. These risk groups are similar throughout the world, but their relative proportions have great geographic variation, both within the United States and worldwide. In the United States and most

Table 1-2. Cumulative reported AIDS cases in adults in the United States according to race or ethnicity through November 1989

Racial or ethnic group	No. of cases	Percent of cases
White, non-Hispanic	64,193	56.7
Black, non-Hispanic	30,487	26.9
Hispanic	17,408	15.4
Asian/Pacific Islander	696	0.6
Native American	152	0.1
Total	113,211	100

Table 1-3. Cumulative reported AIDS cases in adults (≥13 years old) in the United States according to exposure category through November 1989

Exposure category	No. of cases	Percent of cases
Male homosexual or bisexual contact	68,567	60.6
IV drug use	23,722	21.0
IV drug use and male homosexual or bisexual contact	7,923	7.0
Hemophilia or other coagulation disorder	1,047	0.9
Heterosexual contact		
Domestic heterosexual exposure	3,854	3.4
Born in "pattern II" country (see text)	1,603	1.4
Recipient of blood, blood components, tissue, or organs	2,768	2.4
Other or undetermined	3,727	3.3
Total	113,211	100

industrialized countries, homosexual and bisexual men constitute the largest group, followed by heterosexual intravenous (IV) drug users and then by homosexual male IV drug users. In North America, IV drug use as an independent risk factor has been relatively uncommon outside several eastern metropolitan areas, probably reflecting the reduced mobility of drug users compared with that of most homosexual and bisexual men. In addition, there may be regional differences in the frequency with which injection equipment is shared.

The risk categorization of cases has shifted over time. From the early years of the epidemic (1981–1984) to the period from December 1988 through November 1989, the proportion of cases attributed to homosexual male contact declined from 69 to 57 percent; cases in heterosexual IV drug users rose from 16 to 23 percent; and cases attributed to heterosexual acquisition (among persons born in the United States) rose from less than 1 percent to 4.4 percent.[1, 2] Part of these trends may be artifactual, the result of changes in the case definition which enhanced reporting of cases among IV drug users more than cases in homosexuals and bisexuals.

Persons with hemophilia and other coagulation disorders who require repeated treatment with blood products constitute only 0.9 percent of AIDS cases. There are, however, only about 15,000 such individuals in the country, and among these, about 7 percent have acquired AIDS and at least 60 percent are infected with HIV.[1, 2] Thus, on a population basis, persons with hemophilia may be the group at highest risk of acquiring AIDS in the United States.

Persons who received blood transfusions between 1978 and mid-1985 account for 4 percent of AIDS cases nationally. In contrast to the hemophiliacs, however, more than 25 million persons received blood transfusions during this interval, so the actual risk among transfusion recipients was very low. Current blood-banking procedures, including voluntary self-exclusion of persons at risk for AIDS and universal testing of prospective donors for evidence of HIV infection, are almost 100 percent reliable in excluding infected donors. However, persons infected by blood, blood products, and organ transplantation before 1985 will continue to develop AIDS for many years.

Since 1981, 4.8 percent of cases of AIDS in adults have been attributed to heterosexual acquisition of HIV.[2, 4] Persons in this category have been divided into two subcategories: (1) persons from countries where heterosexual exposure is the dominant mode of infection ("pattern II" countries, according to the classification of the World Health Organization) and (2) persons with domestic sexual exposure to a person at increased risk for HIV transmission. As a proportion of all AIDS cases, persons in the latter subcategory are increasing.[2, 4] However, the proportion of cases attributed to domestic heterosexual acquisition may be inflated by persons who deny (or fail to recognize) that they belong to other risk groups. Most women with sexually acquired AIDS in North America are sexual partners of infected IV drug users.

The occurrence of AIDS in persons with no identified risk factor sometimes has been cited as evidence for transmission of HIV by nonintimate personal contact. However, most of the no-identified-risk cases were so classified because there was incomplete information about risk.[1, 2] Studies by the CDC and others have shown that the majority of these patients belonged to, but nonetheless denied connection with, other established risk groups. Because the most common risk factors are viewed negatively by much of society, such denial is to be expected. In other cases, patients were unaware of known risk factors, as might occur if a woman had a sexual relationship with a man who, unknown to her, was bisexual or used IV drugs and shared injection equipment.

Among the 1947 children with AIDS diagnosed through November 1989, 80 percent were born to women at risk and acquired infection in utero or perinatally. Eleven percent of the children with AIDS acquired HIV by transfusion or organ transplantation; 5 percent were hemophiliacs or had similar coagulation disorders; and the remaining 3 percent had no identified risk. As for adults, information was lacking for most of those with no identified risk, and for others the parents are believed to have had risks that were denied.[1, 2]

PREVALENCE OF HIV INFECTION

Numerous studies have been conducted to assess the prevalence of HIV infection in various populations without overt AIDS.[1, 5] Interpretation of nearly all these surveys has been hampered because the persons studied were not entirely representative of the population. For example, most studies of homosexual and bisexual men have involved volunteers for research studies or people who sought HIV serologic testing for personal reasons or for medical diagnosis. Data from prospective blood donors and from most military personnel and recruits exclude persons who admit to homosexual activity, illicit drug use, and other risk factors for AIDS. Nonetheless, these studies have contributed to an understanding of the broad outlines of HIV infection and risk.

Homosexual and bisexual men

More than 75 surveys of homosexual and bisexual men have been conducted in the United States, demonstrating prevalences from 10 to 70 percent; in most studies, the prevalence was 20 to 50 percent.[1, 5] In most settings, higher prevalences have been documented among gay men attending sexually transmitted disease (STD) clinics than among those attending voluntary HIV testing and counseling centers. In San Francisco, 10–20 percent of gay men may have acquired HIV each year from 1980 to 1982, whereas more recent studies suggest that the current annual risk is less than 2 percent. Qualitatively similar trends probably have occurred in most urban areas of the country.

IV Drug users

Many surveys also have examined IV drug users and have documented HIV seroprevalences ranging from zero to 70 percent.[1, 5] The highest prevalences have been found in the east coast cities that contribute most AIDS cases among IV drug users. In most other areas, 5–15 percent of this population have been seropositive. Most of the subjects in these studies were enrolled in drug rehabilitation programs and therefore are highly selected; it has been estimated that only 10–20 percent of IV drug users are in such programs.

Hemophiliacs

Studies in hemophiliacs have shown HIV seroprevalences ranging from 15 percent to almost 90 percent.[1, 5] The highest prevalences have been found in patients with severe hemophilia, which increases the frequency of exposure to clotting factor concentrates and transfused blood. Persons treated with cryoprecipitated factor VIII have had somewhat lower prevalences of HIV infection than those treated with pooled factor VIII concentrates, which are derived from more donors than is the cryoprecipitated product. The overall prevalence of HIV infection in hemophiliacs in the United States probably is more than 50 percent and may be as high as 70 percent. Current blood donation screening practices and pasteurization of clotting factor concentrates have prevented new infections in this population since 1985.

STD Clinics

Studies have been undertaken in a few STD clinic populations to estimate the prevalence of HIV infection in heterosexually active persons without a history of male homosexual contact and IV drug use. Most of these surveys have documented prevalences of zero to 1 percent.[1, 4, 5] A study in a Baltimore, Maryland, STD clinic, which serves a predominantly black population with a high rate of illicit drug use, found prevalences of 2.7 percent and 1.8 percent among men and women, respectively, who denied having risk factors for AIDS.[6] However, this study used anonymous questionnaires to assess risk status, and it is likely that some subjects falsely denied IV drug use, homosexuality, or other risk factors.

Blood donors, military personnel, and hospital admissions

Several populations have been surveyed to assess the prevalence of HIV infection in the "general population," including prospective blood donors, military personnel and recruits, and patients admitted to selected general hospitals.[1, 5] The prevalence of HIV infection in volunteer blood donors is extremely low. In blood donation programs administered nationally by the American Red Cross, the prevalence of HIV infection declined from 0.035 percent in 1985 to 0.015 percent in 1987, and prevalences substantially lower than these have been documented in selected locales. In several studies, more than 75 percent of HIV-infected prospective blood donors had traditional risk factors that had been denied or were unrecognized at the time of donation.

Several million civilian applicants for military service have been tested for HIV antibody, with an overall seroprevalence rate of approximately 0.15 percent. This rate has declined modestly since routine screening began in 1985, especially among white men. Prevalence rates have been two or three times higher in men than in women, and rates in blacks and Hispanics have been several times higher than those in white recruits. There is wide geographic variation in seroprevalence, which tends to parallel the distribution of reported AIDS cases. Although civilians are asked to not apply for military service if they are homosexually active or have used IV drugs, many of these infected applicants nevertheless belong to recognized risk groups. In addition, an unknown proportion may have acquired infection through heterosexual exposure. It is not known whether the declining HIV seroprevalence in recruits is due to stabilization of the risk of HIV infection or to the fact that fewer homosexually active men and IV drug users are now applying for military service. In any case, these data and the stable or declining seroprevalence among blood donors suggest that HIV is not spreading rapidly into populations that lack the traditional risk factors.[1, 5]

Preliminary analysis of surveys of randomly selected patients admitted to 21 hospitals in 19 metropolitan areas indicates HIV seroprevalence rates ranging from 0.02 to 3.4 percent, with a median of 0.6 percent. Not unexpectedly, the seroprevalence was higher in blacks than in whites, and the overall male: female ratio of seropositive patients was 2.8:1.

Several attempts have been made to estimate the number of HIV-infected persons in the United States. Considering the prevalence of HIV infection in various populations, estimating the number of persons with known risk characteristics, and retrograde extrapolation from reported AIDS cases using estimates of the rate of progression from HIV infection to AIDS, the CDC estimates this number to be 1.0 to 1.5 million.[1, 2] In order to estimate this number more accurately, design and assess control strategies, and monitor the HIV epidemic, the CDC is sponsoring standardized HIV seroprevalence surveys in 30 metropolitan areas throughout the country. The study populations include apparently healthy newborn infants and clients of STD clinics, drug rehabilitation programs, reproductive health clinics, and tuberculosis clinics.

TRANSMISSION OF HIV

The modes of transmission of HIV (Table 1-4) may be surmised in general terms from knowledge of the risk groups. All available information on HIV transmission comes from epidemiologic studies, because animal models are of limited usefulness. HIV is present in high concentrations in the semen and blood of infected persons and in lesser concentrations in genital secretions of women. It is present infrequently and in much lower concentrations in urine, saliva, tears, and breast milk.

Sexual transmission

Several studies have documented that receptive anal intercourse carries the highest risk of HIV acquisition for homosexually active men.[1, 7] Practices that lead to rectal injury, such as receptive anal-manual contact ("fisting") and perhaps rectal douching, appear to increase the risk of transmission.

Table 1-4. Modes of transmission of human immunodeficiency virus

Sexual contact
- Intercourse (vaginal, anal)
- Oral-genital contact
- Other

Blood-borne transmission
- Transfusion, blood products
- IV drug use with sharing of injection equipment
- Trauma (health care personnel)
- Cutaneous contact (rare; probably requires epithelial disruption)

In utero and perinatal transmission

Organ or tissue transplantation, therapeutic donor insemination

Nursing (breast milk)

Receptive anal intercourse also appears to be the most risky sexual behavior for women, but vaginal intercourse also is a well-documented mode of acquisition. A history of bleeding after vaginal intercourse also appears to be associated with enhanced risk of infection, suggesting that trauma or other causes of mucosal disruption may be important in transmission.[7]

Numerous studies suggest that the insertive partner in either anal or vaginal intercourse has a lower risk of acquiring HIV from an infected partner than the receptive partner. However, the epidemic of HIV infection in heterosexual men in equatorial Africa and the occurrence of HIV infection in male sexual partners of infected women in industrialized countries leave no doubt that the insertive partner can be infected.[7, 8] The enhanced risk associated with receptive compared with insertive intercourse seems reasonable, because infected secretions are directly deposited into the rectum and vagina. In addition, some data suggest that other STDs that are dependent on transmission to and from mucosal surfaces (e.g., gonorrhea and chlamydial infection) are more efficiently transmitted from men to women than the reverse.

It has been difficult to document that sexual practices other than vaginal intercourse or anal sexual practices are unsafe. A few anecdotal reports suggest that the receptive (oral) partner in fellatio may acquire HIV, especially if there is intraoral ejaculation. Kissing and other forms of sexual expression have not been definitively documented as modes of transmission. However, most people participate in several sexual practices, and the risks of anal and vaginal intercourse might statistically overwhelm those of other activities. Accordingly, it is believed that any sexual contact that allows infected secretions or blood to be deposited into any body cavity, under the skin, or into the bloodstream carries a risk of virus transmission.[1, 7]

Despite the importance of sexual contact as the most common mode of

HIV transmission worldwide, in most circumstances the actual efficiency of sexual transmission appears to be low, and not all steady partners of infected persons become infected themselves. Among 150 female sexual partners of HIV-infected men in San Francisco, only 34 (23 percent) were infected.[9] The prevalence of infection rose from 13 percent of women with 50 or fewer episodes of sexual intercourse with their infected partners to 40 percent of those with 600 or more exposures. Similarly, transmission has not occurred among some homosexual male couples in which an infected and an uninfected partner participated in a full range of sexual practices for several years. On the other hand, it is clear that HIV is sometimes transmitted by a single exposure.

Several factors independent of sexual behaviors appear to enhance the efficiency of sexual transmission or acquisition of HIV. As discussed in Chap. 2, these reported risk factors include the presence of other STDs (especially genital or anorectal ulcerative diseases), the absence of circumcision, and advanced HIV infection with reduced CD4 lymphocyte counts.[7–11]

Limited data suggest other possible risk factors for HIV transmission.[7] Chlamydial infection has been associated with HIV infection in prostitutes in Kenya and Zaire, and vaginal trichomoniasis has been associated with HIV infection in prostitutes in Zaire. It is possible that any genital inflammation enhances transmission in the same manner as genital ulcer disease. One study suggests that the use of oral contraceptive pills is associated with HIV seropositivity in Africa, but these data are controversial and require confirmation (see Chap. 2).

It is probable that variations in the prevalence of risk factors for transmission, as well as differences in sexual behavior, partly explain the geographic variations in the epidemiology of HIV (see Chap. 2). Thus, high frequencies of genital ulcer disease and other STDs in equatorial Africa, differences in the frequency of circumcision, and other factors (e.g., immunodeficiency due to poor nutritional status or other infections) may influence the potential for sustained sexual transmission of the virus. Although sustained heterosexual transmission of HIV appears to be uncommon in most of North America, populations with the potential for sustained heterosexual transmission exist in most industrialized cities. These populations consist primarily of ethnic minorities of low socioeconomic level, with high levels of illicit drug use, prostitution, and STDs.

Transmission via blood and blood products in the United States

Following sexual transmission, exposure to blood or blood products is the next most common mechanism of HIV transmission. Blood transfusion is the most efficient of all modes of transmission, with nearly 100 percent of persons exposed by this route becoming infected.[12] Transmission by sharing of injection equipment among IV drug users, the second most common route of exposure in the United States, is presumed to occur with substantially less efficiency, probably because the inoculum of HIV is smaller than that with transfusion.

There is a small but definite risk of HIV infection among health care workers who sustain accidental parenteral exposure to HIV, most commonly by injury with contaminated needles or other sharp instruments. In a collaborative study conducted by the CDC, among 1031 health care workers with such exposure who were followed for 6 months or longer, 4 (0.4 percent; 95 percent confidence interval, zero to 0.9 percent) were HIV seropositive following exposure; in 3 of these, seroconversion was documented. No seroconversions occurred among 141 persons exposed by contact of their mucous membranes (e.g., mouth, conjunctivae) with contaminated blood or secretions. Three cases of infection in health care workers have been reported following nonparenteral contact with contaminated blood. In each case, the exposure involved prolonged contamination or exposure of cutaneous inflammatory lesions. Moreover, these persons failed to follow standard recommended practices to reduce the occupational risk of infection. Among health care workers without known occupational exposures, the frequencies of HIV infection and reported AIDS apparently are no higher than those in the general population. Nonetheless, the documented cases confirm the need to handle sharp instruments with care and to avoid direct contact with any secretions or blood (see Chap. 14).

Perinatal transmission in the United States

The precise timing of perinatal transmission of HIV to the fetus or newborn is unclear; transplacental transmission and blood exposure during delivery both are plausible. The risk of postnatal exposure (e.g., through breast milk) remains undefined. The efficiency of perinatal transmission is uncertain, partly because there has been no readily available means to distinguish maternal HIV antibody from that produced by the neonate, and because few studies using virus culture, the polymerase chain reaction, or other methods to detect HIV or its antigens have been reported to date. Most authorities estimate that 20–50 percent of children born to infected mothers in the United States acquire HIV (see Chap. 10).

Other modes of transmission

HIV has been transmitted by therapeutic donor insemination, and several cases of infection by transplantation of contaminated organs or tissues have been documented. All potential semen or organ donors must be screened for HIV infection. Although a few cases of transmission by breast milk have been reported, this appears to be rare. In industrialized countries, infected mothers are advised to avoid nursing their infants. In developing countries, however, the nutritional and immunologic benefits of nursing are believed to outweigh the risk of HIV transmission (see Chaps. 2 and 10).

There is strong epidemiologic evidence that HIV transmission does not occur with detectable frequency by nonintimate contact with infected persons, despite the fact that HIV can be shown to survive on inanimate objects. One study involved 101 members of households containing persons with AIDS or other forms of HIV infection.[13] None were sexual partners or shared drug injection equipment with the infected persons. The duration of contact with the infected persons ranged from 3 months to 4 years, with a median of 22 months. The only household member found to be infected was a young child of a mother with AIDS; the child was believed to have acquired HIV at or near the time of birth. No other persons were infected despite high frequencies of sharing kitchens, toilet facilities, and drinking or eating utensils, and occasional sharing of toothbrushes and razors. Other studies have involved more than 400 household contacts, with no documented HIV transmissions.

Some persons have expressed fear that mosquitoes or other blood-feeding arthropods might transmit HIV. However, the absence of infection in household contacts in geographic areas where mosquitoes are prevalent (e.g., equatorial Africa, southern Florida) indicates that arthropod-borne transmission occurs extremely rarely, if ever. Although theoretically there may be other, unrecognized modes of transmission of HIV, they must be exceedingly rare.[14]

REFERENCES

1. Curran JW, Jaffe HW, Hardy AM, et al. Epidemiology of HIV infection and AIDS in the United States. *Science* 1988;239:610–616.
2. Centers for Disease Control. Update: acquired immunodeficiency syndrome–United States, 1981–1988. *MMWR* 1989;38:229–236.
3. Karon JM, Dondero TJ, Curran JW. The projected incidence of AIDS and estimated prevalence of HIV infection in the United States. *J AIDS* 1988;1:542–550.
4. Centers for Disease Control. Update: Heterosexual transmission of AIDS and HIV infection—United States. *MMWR* 1989;38:423–434.
5. Centers for Disease Control. AIDS and human immunodeficiency virus infection in the United States: 1988 update. *MMWR* 1989;38:1–38.

6. Quinn TC, Glasser D, Cannon RO, et al. Human immunodeficiency virus infection among patients attending clinics for sexually transmitted diseases. *N Engl J Med* 1988;318:197–203.

7. Holmberg SD, Horsburgh CR Jr, Ward JW, Jaffe HW. Biologic factors in the sexual transmission of human immunodeficiency virus. *J Infect Dis* 1989;160:116–125.

8. Quinn TC, Piot P, McCormick JB, et al. Serologic and immunologic studies in patients with AIDS in North America and Africa. *JAMA* 1987;257:2617–2621.

9. Padian N, Shiboski S. Heterogenous male-to-female transmission of human immunodeficiency virus [abstract T.A.O.16]. Fifth International Conference on AIDS, Montreal, June 4–9, 1989.

10. Simonsen JN, Cameron DW, Gakinya MN, et al. Human immunodeficiency virus infection among men with sexually transmitted diseases: Experience from a center in Africa. *N Engl J Med* 1988;319:274–278.

11. Stamm WE, Handsfield HH, Rompalo AM, Ashley RL, Roberts PL, Corey L. The association between genital ulcer disease and acquisition of HIV in homosexual men. *JAMA* 1988;260:1429–1433.

12. Berglund O, Beckman S, Grillner L, et al. HIV transmission by blood transfusions in Stockholm 1979–1985: Nearly uniform transmission from infected donors. *AIDS* 1988;2:51–54.

13. Friedland GH, Saltzman BR, Rogers MF, et al. Lack of transmission of HTLV-III/LAV infection to household contacts of patients with AIDS or AIDS-related complex with oral candidiasis. *N Engl J Med* 1986;314:344–349.

14. Lifson AR. Do alternate modes for transmission of human immunodeficiency virus exist? A review. *JAMA* 1988;259:1353–1356.

2

Global Patterns of HIV Infection: Implications for the Clinician

Joan Kreiss
Ann M. Kimball
King K. Holmes

GLOBAL INCIDENCE OF AIDS AND PATTERNS OF TRANSMISSION OF HIV

When a clinician sees a patient from another country or one who has traveled to another country, some knowledge about the epidemiology of HIV and its transmission pattern in that country is essential to estimate the risk of HIV. As of September 1, 1989, 178,000 cases of AIDS had been reported to the World Health Organization (WHO). Because reporting is far from complete, it is estimated that over 500,000 cases of AIDS had occurred worldwide by mid-1989, with perhaps 5 to 10 million people infected by HIV. Assuming no vaccine, drug therapy, or major behavioral change, it has been estimated that the cumulative number of HIV infections worldwide by the year 2000 will be about 20 million.

On a global basis, the vast majority of HIV infections are sexually transmitted. Four patterns of transmission have been described by WHO.[1] In the industrialized countries of North America, Western Europe, Australia, and New Zealand, 80–90 percent of the cases of AIDS and HIV infection are attributable to homosexual contact among men or to IV drug use; this is referred to as pattern I. In sub-Saharan Africa and in certain Caribbean countries (e.g., Haiti, the Dominican Republic), transmission is predominantly heterosexual, referred to as pattern II. In some Latin American countries (e.g., Brazil), both heterosexual and homosexual transmission are common; the pattern is evolving from pattern I to pattern II, referred to as pattern I/II. Pattern III refers to areas where HIV infection is still uncommon (e.g., China, North Africa) and where the predominant modes of transmission have not yet been established. HIV-1 is implicated in almost all cases of AIDS in North America, Europe, Latin America, Australia, and Asia, and is epidemic in Central, East, and Southern Africa. HIV-2 is widespread only in West Africa, where its highest prevalence has been found in prostitutes, and therefore is also probably spread by heterosexual transmission. HIV-2 differs from HIV-1 over a substantial proportion of its genome (see Chap. 5). It is now accepted that HIV-2, like HIV-1, causes AIDS, although the rate of progression to AIDS may be lower with HIV-2 infection.

Antibodies to HIV-1 were first detected in a blood specimen collected in Central Africa in 1959. The first cases of AIDS were identified, in retrospect, in the mid-1970s in Central Africa, where HIV-1 has spread quickly, mainly by heterosexual contact. Perinatal transmission of HIV-1 is also common in Africa, as is transmission by blood transfusion. Transmission by unsterile injection equipment has also been implicated, but transmission by IV drug use and male homosexual contract have been uncommon in Africa. By now, 10–20 percent or more of the young adult population of some cities in Zaire, Rwanda, Uganda, Zambia, Malawi, the Congo, and Tanzania have been infected, and the epidemic has spread progressively to East, West, and Southern Africa.[2] HIV infection has been much more prevalent in the urban centers and interurban corridors of Africa than in the rural areas. Its prevalence has been extraordinarily high in hospitalized adult and pediatric patients in some areas of Africa (e.g., 37 percent of hospitalized patients and 53 percent of outpatients in a survey of 15 hospitals in Uganda),[3] indicating the extent to which HIV infection now influences the character of clinical practice in such settings. The epidemic of AIDS has spread with alarming rapidity in many countries in sub-Saharan Africa. In the Ivory Coast, where AIDS was first recognized as recently as 1985, 43 percent of patients in a major hospital in Abidjan were infected with HIV, and 33 percent of hospital deaths were attributable to AIDS by late 1988.[4] The distribution of HIV-1 and HIV-2 in Africa is shown in Fig. 2-1. The prevalence of infection in healthy populations, including blood donors, hospital workers, and pregnant women, is shown in Table 2-1 for selected cities in Africa and Latin America.

Two-thirds of the cases of AIDS reported to the WHO have been reported from the Americas, and 84 percent of the cases from that region have been reported from the United States. AIDS has been reported by all countries in the Western Hemisphere. The incidence of reported AIDS cases for 1988 was 13 per million for Latin America, 72 per million for the Caribbean, and 106 per million for North America.

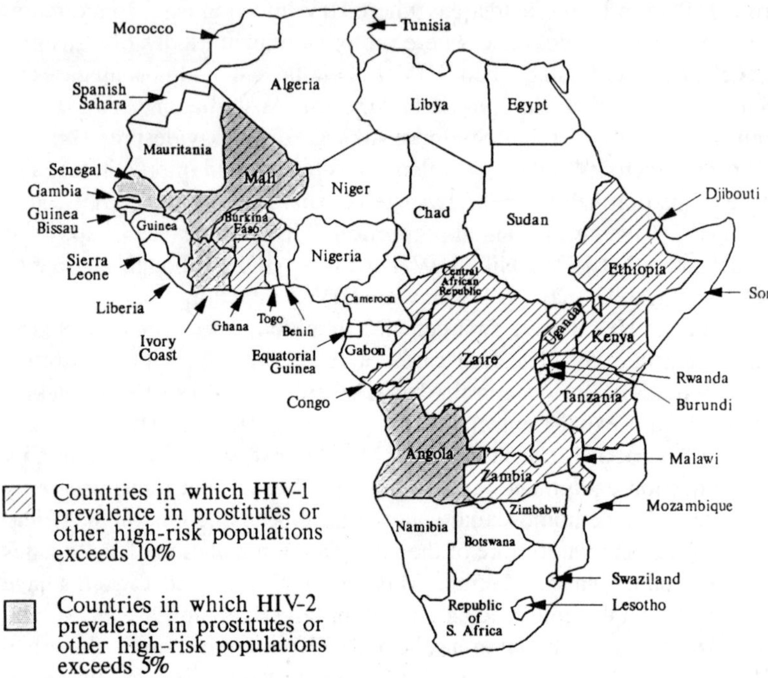

Figure 2-1. Distribution of HIV-1 and HIV-2 infection in African countries.

The great majority of the cases of AIDS reported in the Americas are attributed to infection with HIV through homosexual or heterosexual activity.[5] The region has countries that fit patterns I, II, or I/II. In no country is AIDS currently believed to be solely an imported phenomenon. At this time in the Caribbean subregion, including Haiti and the Dominican Republic, transmission of HIV occurs primarily through heterosexual contact or through vertical transmission from mother to child. Homosexual and bisexual transmission predominate in most of the remaining countries of the Americas. Many cases in Latin America involve bisexual men (15–20 percent), who often have stable heterosexual relationships as well. In Central America the ratio of male:female cases has been declining, as heterosexual transmission apparently is becoming increasingly important.

In Asia, patterns of spread are not yet clearly defined, although in Thailand the prevalence of HIV in IV drug users has risen rapidly over the past 2 years, and there are recent reports of rapidly increasing rates in prostitutes in Bangkok and Cheng Mei, Thailand, and in parts of India.

Table 2-1. Prevalence of HIV antibody in blood donors, hospital workers, and pregnant women in selected cities in Africa and Latin America

Location	Blood donors %	(year)	Hospital workers %	(year)	Pregnant women %	(year)
Africa						
Kampala, Uganda	16	(1986–1987)	NA		24	(1989)
Nairobi, Kenya	NA		NA		4	(1988)
Lusaka, Zambia	18	(1985)	19	(1985)	9	(1985)
Blantyre, Malawi	NA		NA		19	(1988)
Mbeya, Tanzania	10	(1989)	NA		11	(1989)
Kigali, Rwanda	18	(1985)	19	(1985)	29	(1988–1989)
Kinshasa, Zaire	9	(1986)	9	(1986)	6	(1986–1987)
Brazzaville, Congo	NA		NA		4	(1988–1989)
Abidjan, Ivory Coast*	9	(1988)	NA		9	(1989)
Dakar, Senegal*	1.5	(1988)	0.6	(1987)	0.3	(1988)
Latin America and the Caribbean						
Panama City, Panama	0.2	(1986)	NA		NA	
7 cities, Columbia	0.1	(1987)	NA		NA	
Buenos Aires, Argentina	0.25	(1988)	NA		NA	
Mexico City, Mexico	0.7	(1986–1987)	NA		NA	
Puebla City, Mexico	0.7	(1985–1986)	NA		NA	
Rio de Janeiro, Brazil	0.2	(1985–1987)	NA		NA	
São Paulo, Brazil	0.2	(1985–1986)	NA		NA	
Santos, Brazil	NA		NA		3.5	(1988)
Port au Prince, Haiti	NA		NA		10.5	(1988)

Note: NA = not available.

*Combined prevalence of HIV-1 or HIV-2 infection in Ivory Coast and Senegal.

HETEROSEXUAL TRANSMISSION OF HIV IN DEVELOPING COUNTRIES

Spread of HIV-1 in Africa has been fostered by rapid population growth, rural-urban migration, disintegration of traditional cultures, and other factors contributing to prostitution and heterosexual promiscuity.[6] Heterosexual transmission accounts for the vast majority of HIV infections in adults in Africa and in the Caribbean. In the United States, heterosexual transmission accounts for a small but growing proportion of cases of AIDS (4–5 percent of all cases, 20–30 percent of the cases in women). Thus, the ratio of males to females with AIDS is approximately 1:1 in Africa versus greater than

10:1 in industrialized countries. In an initial study of HIV infection in Rwanda, 69 percent of cases occurred in prostitutes or heterosexually promiscuous men or their wives. In subsequent studies, prostitutes have been found to be at high risk, particularly in Africa (Table 2-2). The prevalence of serum antibody to HIV has been increasing rapidly among prostitutes throughout the developing world, despite efforts in some areas to protect prostitutes and their customers by promoting condom use. In a slum area of Nairobi, the prevalence of HIV infection rose rapidly from 4 percent to over 85 percent during a 4- to 5-year period.[7] The risk of transmission to and from prostitutes seems to vary in relation to the number of clients, use of condoms, and presence of risk factors, as discussed later. In Asia the prevalence of HIV-1 has been low in most prostitute groups but has begun to increase rapidly in certain groups of prostitutes in India and Thailand, perhaps heralding an increasing risk of heterosexual transmission in these regions. In the United States the prevalence of antibody in prostitutes also varies greatly, but this appears to be more often attributable to patterns of IV drug use than to sexual transmission.

Studies of African men attending STD clinics—many of whom have had sexual contact with prostitutes—also demonstrate that prostitutes and their contacts are important reservoirs and disseminators of infection on that continent. Antibody to HIV was found in 12 percent of such men in Nairobi,

Table 2-2. Prevalence of serum antibody to HIV among high-risk groups in Africa and Latin America

Location	Year	Female prostitutes (%)	Male STD clinic attendees (%)
Africa			
Butare, Rwanda	1984	88	28
Nairobi, Kenya	1988–1989	85	12
Kampala, Uganda	1987	NA	36
Bukoba, Tanzania	1986	37	NA
Addis Ababa, Ethiopa	1988	19	12
Kinshasa, Zaire	1988–1989	37	NA
Lusaka, Zambia	1985	NA	27
Dakar, Senegal	1989	12*	NA
Various cities, the Gambia	1988	26*	NA
Latin America and the Caribbean			
Port au Prince, Haiti	1988	42	NA
Buenos Aires, Argentina	1988	6	NA

Note: NA = not available.

*Predominantly HIV-2 in Senegal and the Gambia.

Kenya, and Addis Ababa, Ethiopia, and in 27–28 percent in Butare, Rwanda, and Lusaka, Zambia (Table 2-2). A prospective study of risk of female-to-male transmission involved 293 seronegative men coming to a Nairobi STD clinic within 4 weeks after sexual exposure to a group of prostitutes, most of whom had HIV infection. The cumulative frequency of HIV seroconversion among the exposed men over the next several months was 18 percent![8] This extraordinary rate of female-to-male transmission is much higher than was previously estimated from most studies in the United States.

Risk factors for sexual transmission

Why is heterosexual transmission so much more important in Africa and the Caribbean than in developed countries? Answers may include differences in heterosexual behavior, including a greater frequency of prostitution in Africa and the high frequency of risk factors that facilitate sexual transmission. These risk factors are summarized in Table 2-3. Five studies in Kenya have found that genital ulcer disease is correlated with increased risk of HIV infection in heterosexuals. In a cohort of seronegative Nairobi prostitutes, the odds of seroconversion were three times higher among those with genital

Table 2-3. Risk factors that have been repeatedly implicated in the sexual transmission of HIV

Probability of sexual exposure to HIV
- Prevalence of HIV in various risk groups
- Choice of sexual partner from high-risk group
- Number of sexual partners
- Number of episodes of intercourse

Sexual practices
- Receptive anorectal intercourse (male or female) >> receptive vaginal intercourse > insertive rectal or vaginal intercourse*

STDs
- Genital and anorectal ulcer disease: chancroid, HSV-2, syphilis, *Chlamydia trachomatis* infection

Circumcision status
- Presence of a foreskin is a risk factor for men

Stage of infection in sexual partner
- Low CD4 lymphocyte count

*It is possible but not yet clearly proven that receptive vaginal intercourse is riskier than insertive vaginal intercourse.

ulcers (usually chancroid) during follow-up than among those who remained free of genital ulcers. Of men presenting to the Nairobi STD clinic soon after intercourse with prostitutes,[9] the subsequent risk of seroconversion was nearly five times greater among those with genital ulcers than among those with urethritis. Genital ulcers may provide portals through which HIV may be shed or inoculated. Mononuclear cells at the base of a genital ulcer may shed virus or be especially susceptible if exposed to HIV. The fact that chancroid, syphilis, and genital herpes are epidemic throughout many African countries may help to explain the epidemic of heterosexually transmitted HIV in Africa.

Recent epidemics of chancroid and syphilis have also been observed in poor urban black and Hispanic populations in the United States in association with prostitution and illicit drug use (especially crack cocaine); the possibility that genital ulcer disease may have a significant impact on the heterosexual spread of HIV in the developed world, as well as in the developing world, is of real concern. Other STDs, such as *Chlamydia trachomatis* infection of the cervix, may also facilitate sexual transmission of HIV, perhaps by causing genital inflammation and microulcerations. It is possible that any genital inflammation represents a risk factor for heterosexual transmission of HIV and that proctitis of any cause represents a risk factor for acquisition by receptive anorectal intercourse.

The importance of other STDs as cofactors in the transmission of HIV is also assumed but not well documented in some areas of the Caribbean and Latin America. Reported rates of STDs are several times higher for the Caribbean than for the countries of the southern cone of South America (Chile, Uruguay, Argentina, Paraguay) and may contribute to the greater frequency of heterosexual transmission in the Caribbean.

Many studies indicate that receptive anorectal intercourse is a significant risk factor for acquisition of HIV infection by either gender. Lack of circumcision was found to be an important risk factor for HIV acquisition in men in the prospective study of men in Nairobi mentioned previously (more than an eightfold higher risk compared to circumcised men after sexual exposure to prostitutes), and similar findings have been reported from Miami. A close negative correlation has been found between the distribution of circumcision practices in Africa and the distribution of HIV-1 infection, supporting the hypothesis that patterns of circumcision may partially explain differing rates of spread of the HIV epidemic in different countries or ethnic groups.

Oral contraceptive use was associated with an increased risk of HIV infection in Kenyan prostitutes—a controversial finding which has yet to be assessed in other settings. The prevalence of HIV infection in Kinshasa, Zaire, and the percentage of AIDS cases, has been three to four times higher in young women than in young men (Fig. 2-2). While this may well be related to gender differences in sexual behavior, it is possible that young women are particularly susceptible to HIV infection—perhaps because of the high prevalence of cervical ectopy in young women.

In early studies in the United States of stable couples in which one member had acquired HIV infection through clotting factor concentrate or blood transfusions, the rate of either female-to-male or male-to-female transmission was only 10–20 percent, even after years of sexual exposure. However, the risk of heterosexual transmission evidently becomes greater as the peripheral blood CD4 lymphocyte count decreases, an observation that has now been confirmed in partner studies. This is consistent with an increasing prevalence of circulating free virus in plasma as the infection progresses. Thus, differences in observed rates of heterosexual transmission could be related to the stage of HIV infection in the index case. If the HIV epidemic is of longer duration in Central Africa than elsewhere, this could contribute to the greater efficiency today of heterosexual transmission in Central Africa.

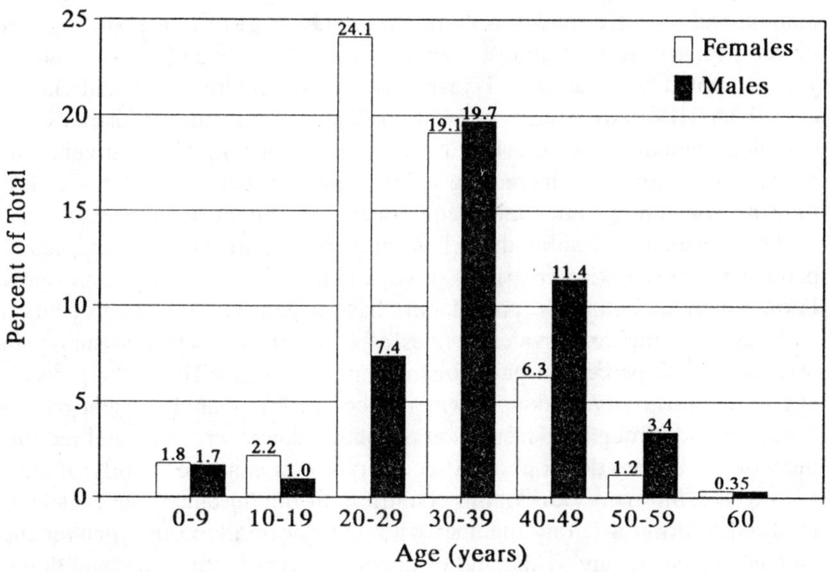

Figure 2-2. Distribution by age and sex of the first 500 AIDS cases diagnosed in Kinshasa, Zaire, between August 1985 and December 1985.[9] Females were significantly younger than males. Women accounted for the majority of AIDS cases in the 20–29 age group, whereas men accounted for the majority of cases in the 40–49 and 50–59 age groups.

TRANSMISSION OF HIV BY BLOOD TRANSFUSION IN DEVELOPING COUNTRIES

From the "look-back" program in this country, which traces recipients of infected blood products administered before HIV screening was available, it appears that receipt of a contaminated unit of blood is associated with a 90 percent or higher risk of infection. In the United States, where all donated blood is screened for HIV antibody, the current prevalence of that antibody is about 0.01 percent. However, blood transfusions have been a major mode of transmission of HIV in Africa and Latin America. As shown in Table 2-1, seroprevalence rates in blood donors in certain African cities have been as high as 18 percent. Women have been at particular risk from transfusion because of the frequent administration of blood during pregnancy and childbirth. Further, anemia is common in many developing countries because of nutritional deficiencies, infections such as malaria, and hemoglobinopathies. The relationship between malaria and HIV infection at a major hospital in Kinshasa, Zaire, was studied.[10] In a survey of children admitted to a pediatric ward, 67 percent had malaria and 47 percent received a transfusion during their hospitalization. Chloroquine-resistant falciparum malaria had recently spread to Zaire, and the number of transfusions given on the pediatric service almost doubled from 1984–1985 to 1985–1986. It was estimated that during a 1-year period, 561 children with malaria received an HIV-seropositive blood transfusion. This study illustrates the complex epidemiology of AIDS by demonstrating how the resurgence of malaria, due in part to increasing chloroquine resistance, accelerated HIV transmission through increased requirements for blood transfusions.

The prevalence of antibody to HIV in blood donors has been less than 1 percent in most Latin American surveys (Table 2-1). However, in many Latin American countries, paid donors have been a major source of blood and have had higher prevalence rates of HIV infection. In one survey in Mexico City, 7 percent of paid donors were positive for HIV. The percentage of seropositivity in donors was reduced to less than 1 percent over a 2-year period through the institution of routine donor screening and recruitment of a voluntary donor pool. A second type of donor, the "family" donor, is also used in many developing countries. In this instance, the patient is required to bring a family member who will donate blood in order for the patient to receive care. This kind of donor is less risky than the paid donor but less safe than the strictly voluntary donor, probably due to the tendency of families to pay strangers to serve as family donors if a family member is not available. Thus, from the clinical perspective, anyone who has received blood products in the AIDS epidemic areas of Africa or the Americas since the onset of the HIV epidemics in these areas, including blood recipients before mid-1985 in the United States, is at some risk of having contracted HIV.

PERINATAL TRANSMISSION IN DEVELOPING COUNTRIES

As noted, the female:male sex ratio for AIDS cases during the childbearing years in sub-Saharan Africa is as high as 3:1 (Fig. 2-2). The female:male sex ratio for the prevalence of serum antibody to HIV may be even higher. Because young women represent such a high proportion of HIV carriers, and because birth rates are so high in Africa, vertical transmission of HIV from infected mother to offspring is a major public health problem. Surveys of pregnant women in Africa have yielded HIV antibody prevalence rates as high as 29 percent (Table 2-1).

The risks of congenital, perinatal, and postnatal HIV transmission have not been clearly defined yet. In two hospitals in Kinshasa, Zaire, the risk of vertical transmission varied according to the degree of immunosuppression in the mother, analogous to the effects of immunosuppression on heterosexual transmission, as discussed earlier.[11] HIV was isolated from cord blood from 6 of 18 infants of seropositive women with CD4 cell counts of 400, or less, compared with 0 of 19 infants of women with CD4 cell counts greater than 400.

Postnatal transmission, perhaps by breast-feeding, has been well documented in several cases, particularly where the mother has been acutely infected after birth from blood transfusion. HIV can be isolated from breast milk; however, it has yet to be shown conclusively that breast milk is a common vehicle for transmission. In the West, seropositive mothers are advised to forego breast-feeding. In Africa, where bottle-feeding is associated with appreciable infant morbidity and mortality due to diarrheal disease, HIV-related public health policies regarding breast-feeding must await further information.

IMPLICATIONS OF THE GLOBAL HIV PANDEMIC FOR CLINICIANS

Identification of individuals at risk for HIV infection

The identification of individuals at high risk for HIV infection in the United States and other pattern I countries, where AIDS occurs primarily in homosexual men and IV drug users, is now familiar to most clinicians. Ascertainment of the HIV risk for individuals from pattern II countries, where heterosexual transmission predominates, is more difficult. As discussed, individuals who have had blood transfusions, multiple sexual partners, sex with prostitutes, or STDs (particularly genital ulcerative disease), and men who are uncircumcised, are at increased risk for HIV infection. In areas of high HIV prevalence, however, many heterosexually active adults may acquire HIV infection even in the absence of these specific risk factors, and the threshold for screening such individuals for HIV antibodies, especially in the presence of signs or symptoms possibly attributable to HIV, should be low.

When to suspect HIV-2 infection

Although sporadic HIV-2 infection has been reported in North America, Europe, and Brazil, in epidemic form it remains fairly geographically circumscribed in West Africa. Individuals at possible risk for HIV-2 infection include Africans from Senegal, Guinea-Bissau, Mali, Burkina Faso, Ivory Coast, and Angola (Fig. 2-1), individuals who have had sex with or shared needles with Africans from the HIV-2 endemic areas, and individuals who have traveled to and received blood transfusions in these countries.

There are no distinctive clinical features that allow one to distinguish between HIV-1 and HIV-2 infection in patients with symptomatic disease. If an individual has signs or symptoms suggestive of HIV-related illness and has epidemiologic risk factors for HIV-2, serologic tests for both HIV-1 and HIV-2 should be ordered. There is some cross-reactivity between the two viruses in both ELISA and Western blot assays. The sensitivity of various commercial HIV-1 ELISA assays to detect HIV-2 antibodies ranges from 60 percent to over 90 percent. Individuals with HIV-2 infection may thus have either a positive or a negative HIV-1 ELISA result. The HIV-1 Western blot pattern is most often indeterminate, but it may be negative or positive. Simultaneous reactions to both HIV-1 and HIV-2 by Western blot assay may represent dual infections, but at present this can be confirmed only with virus culture, polymerase chain reaction assays, or virus-specific peptide assays. Most serum samples with dual reactivity that have been further characterized have been found to represent cross-reactivity of HIV-1 antibodies with HIV-2 antigens rather than coinfection with the two viruses.

In the absence of epidemiologic risk factors for HIV-2, HIV-2 serologic testing in an individual from a low-prevalence country such as the United States is likely to be of limited utility, even in a symptomatic individual with an indeterminate HIV-1 Western blot result. The positive predictive value of an HIV-2 Western blot result in this setting would be low, and the majority of positive results would be falsely positive.

Clinical manifestations of HIV infection in relation to the country of origin

Both the frequency and the type of clinical manifestations of AIDS in developing countries have differed considerably from the manifestations seen in developed countries. This is attributable to many factors, including lack of facilities in such countries for diagnosis of certain opportunistic infections (e.g., central nervous system toxoplasmosis, *Pneumocystis carinii* pneumonia [PCP]); delay in diagnosis (the mean duration of symptoms before diagnosis of AIDS averaged 1 year in Kinshasa, Zaire); and true differences in manifestations related to differing prevalences of endemic diseases. Because of limited resources for diagnosis, provisional WHO clinical case definitions for adult and pediatric AIDS have been established for use in developing countries (Table 2-4). The increasing availability

Table 2-4. Provisional WHO clinical case definition for AIDS where diagnostic resources are limited

Adults

AIDS in an adult is defined by the existence of at least two of the major signs associated with at least one minor sign, in the absence of known causes of immunosuppression such as cancer or severe malnutrition or other recognized causes.

Major signs
- Weight loss greater than 10 percent of body weight
- Chronic diarrhea for more than 1 month
- Prolonged fever for more than 1 month (intermittent or constant)

Minor signs
- Persistent cough for more than 1 month
- Generalized pruritic dermatitis
- Recurrent herpes zoster infection
- Oropharyngeal candidiasis
- Chronic progressive and disseminated herpes simplex virus infections
- Generalized lymphadenopathy

The presence of generalized Kaposi's sarcoma or cryptococcal meningitis is sufficient for the diagnosis of AIDS.

Children

Pediatric AIDS is suspected in an infant or child presenting with at least two major signs associated with at least two minor signs in the absence of other known causes of immunosuppression.

Major signs
- Weight loss or abnormally slow growth
- Chronic diarrhea for more than 1 month
- Prolonged fever for more than 1 month

Minor signs
- Generalized lymphadenopathy
- Oropharyngeal candidiasis
- Repeated common infections (otitis, pharyngitis, etc.)
- Persistent cough for more than 1 month
- Generalized dermatitis
- Confirmed maternal HIV infection

of serologic testing for HIV in developing countries will permit serology to complement these clinical criteria for the diagnosis of AIDS. Thus, the Pan American Health Organization has also developed a clinical algorithm for identification of notifiable cases of AIDS based upon serologic testing for HIV and easily identified manifestations of HIV-induced immunosuppression (Fig. 2-3).

Gastrointestinal and dermatologic manifestations have been more common and pulmonary manifestations less common in African patients than in North American patients with AIDS. The most common presentation of AIDS in Central Africa and Haiti has been progressive, extreme weight loss, usually accompanied by chronic diarrhea and fever. In Uganda and Tanzania, this syndrome has been referred to as *slim disease*. Specific gastrointestinal pathogens identified in one-half of those with diarrhea and weight loss in tropical settings include *Cryptosporidium* (which is now becoming less common in homosexual men with AIDS in the United States, perhaps because of changing sexual practices that reduce the risk of transmission of gastrointestinal pathogens), *Isospora belli, Entamoeba histolytica, Strongyloides stercoralis, Giardia lamblia, Salmonella*, and *Mycobacterium*.

Common skin manifestations of HIV infection in the tropics include herpes zoster, prurigo, and—in certain Central African countries—disseminated Kaposi's sarcoma. Prurigo refers to a generalized chronic papular pruritic eruption distributed on the extremities more than on the trunk; severe pruritis leads to excoriation, secondary infection, and hyperpigmentation. Disseminated Kaposi's sarcoma is now seen in heterosexuals with AIDS in those areas of Africa where the classical forms of Kaposi's sarcoma were endemic in the pre-AIDS era (e.g., Uganda, Tanzania, Rwanda, Burundi, Zaire, Zambia).

Other manifestations of HIV infection that have been particularly common in the tropics include oral and esophageal candidiasis, tuberculosis, and cryptococcal meningitis. A review of national data from Brazil suggests that the most common opportunistic infections seen were candidiasis (33 percent), PCP (12 percent), and tuberculosis (11 percent). Among 406 cases in Rio de Janiero, tuberculosis (18 percent) was actually detected more frequently than was PCP (14 percent).[12] However, the diagnosis of PCP is difficult in many areas of the region. In Panama,[13] a review of 31 AIDS cases demonstrated that the most common opportunistic infections were histoplasmosis (5), tuberculosis (4), PCP (4), disseminated candidiasis (4), cytomegaloviral pneumonia (2), and toxoplasmosis (1). The importance of tuberculosis has recently been emphasized in the finding that the majority of tuberculosis patients seen as outpatients in Port au Prince, Haiti, had HIV infection.

Persons from developing countries who present with AIDS in industrialized countries also have distinctive patterns of opportunistic infections

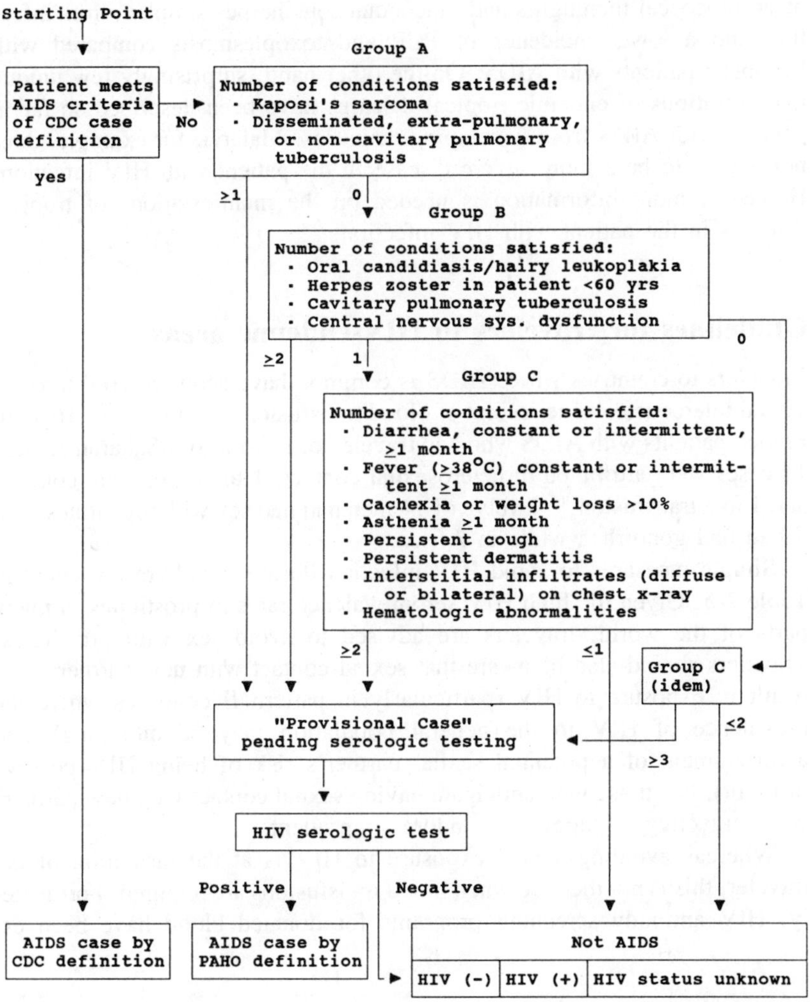

Figure 2-3. Provisional algorithm for identification of cases of AIDS notifiable to the Pan American Health Organization. This approach is based upon a positive serologic diagnosis of HIV infection together with the presence of certain relatively easy-to-diagnose manifestations associated with advanced stages of immunosuppression caused by HIV. (A detailed description is available from Dr. Ann M. Kimball, Pan American Health Organization, 525 23rd St. N.W., Washington, D.C. 20037.)

that reflect the prevalence of endemic, latent opportunistic infections in their country of origin. For example, Haitians presenting with AIDS in the United States often have tuberculosis or central nervous system toxoplasmosis. Africans presenting with AIDS in Western Europe have a higher incidence of cryptococcal meningitis and mucocutaneous herpes simplex virus infection and a lower incidence of PCP and toxoplasmosis compared with European patients with AIDS. On the other hand, surprisingly few unique manifestations of endemic tropical diseases have been described so far in persons with AIDS from developing countries. Malaria, for example, does not appear to be a more severe disease in the patient with HIV infection. However, more information is needed on the manifestations of tropical diseases in the patient with HIV infection.

Guidelines for travelers to HIV-endemic areas

Travelers to countries where AIDS is common have acquired HIV through sexual intercourse or the receipt of blood transfusions. In a study of 16 adult French patients with AIDS who had traveled or lived in sub-Saharan Africa, 14 cases were attributed to heterosexual contact, 1 to homosexual contact, and 1 to a transfusion.[14] Twelve of 14 men had had sex with prostitutes, and 7 had had gonorrhea while in Africa.

Simple measures to avoid HIV infection during travel are presented in Table 2-5. Given the high HIV seroprevalence rates in prostitutes in many parts of the world, travelers are advised to avoid sex with prostitutes. Travelers should also be aware that sexual contact with new partners may result in exposure to HIV (particularly in pattern II countries where the prevalence of HIV in the general population may be quite high and ascertainment of a potential sexual partner's risk of being HIV positive difficult). For those who anticipate having sexual contact with new partners while traveling, a supply of condoms is prudent.

Whereas avoiding sexual exposure to HIV is at the discretion of the traveler, this is not the case when blood transfusions are required. Fortunately, HIV antibody screening programs for donated blood have been es-

Table 2-5. Guidelines for travelers to HIV-endemic areas

1. Avoid high-risk sexual exposure
2. Precautions to reduce the risk of blood transfusion
   - Obtain antimalarial chemoprophylaxis
   - Reduce the risk of trauma
   - Know the blood type of self and fellow travelers
3. Precautions to reduce the risk of medical injection
   - Complete immunization before travel
   - Insist on the use of disposable (sealed package) needle and syringe

tablished in most large urban centers in AIDS-endemic areas. Travelers may take precautions to avoid the potential need for transfusions, such as taking antimalarial chemoprophylaxis where indicated or avoiding driving while intoxicated. Knowledge of one's blood type may be helpful, particularly if a group of tourists is traveling together and a matched low-risk blood donor can be identified from within the group. Travelers who do receive blood transfusions in AIDS-endemic areas may wish to be tested for HIV antibodies when they return home and 3 and 6 months after the transfusion.

The third potential risk for HIV exposure for travelers is through medical injections. From studies of needlestick accidents in health care workers in the United States, it appears that the risk of acquiring HIV infection from a contaminated needle is less than 1 percent. For travelers, even this small risk is largely avoidable. First, individuals who are planning a trip should be aware of the immunization requirements of the countries to be visited and should receive immunization before embarking. Second, persons who require injections while traveling should request that they be administered with an unused (sealed package), disposable needle and syringe. Travelers who will be living for prolonged periods in AIDS-endemic areas and who anticipate a need for injections, such as periodic gamma globulin injections for hepatitis A prophylaxis, may wish to carry a supply of disposable needles and syringes.

Travelers may be reassured that there is no epidemiologic evidence to suggest that HIV transmission occurs through insect vectors, casual contact, food, or water. Finally, travelers from the United States should bear in mind that this country probably has a higher prevalence of HIV infection than most countries they are likely to visit.

IMPACT ON SOCIETY

By 1991 it is predicted that 270,000 persons in the United States will have had AIDS. Costs for direct medical care in 1991 have been projected to be as high as $16 billion. In the developing world, the economic impact will be comparatively greater. In African countries—where the per capita annual health expenditure may be as low as a few dollars—care of HIV-related illness could quickly drain all available health care resources. The AIDS epidemic also may have an adverse impact on other important diseases in developing countries. For example, HIV-infected persons may have an attenuated response to vaccines. As the number of children with perinatal HIV infection grows, herd immunity to diseases such as measles or polio may be reduced sufficiently to allow epidemics to sweep through communities. Furthermore, the natural history of various diseases such as tuberculois, genital herpes, and chancroid is altered in persons with HIV infection. Thus, HIV may increase the transmission of tuberculosis and other communicable diseases.

The economic impact of the AIDS epidemic can be measured not only in health care costs but also in the loss of years of productive life. Worldwide, persons 20–40 years old are at greatest risk for HIV infection. In some African countries, 20 percent or more of young urban adults—a considerable portion of the productive work force—have already been infected with HIV. Because women comprise a high percentage of infected young adults, perinatal transmission will result in substantial infant and childhood mortality in the next generation. Thus, HIV infection already has become firmly entrenched in some populations, both in the present generation and in the next. AIDS has become the number one cause of lost years of productive life in some developing countries.

CONTROL OF THE EPIDEMIC

Global efforts to halt the spread of HIV infection have been planned and are being implemented. In the past few years, government leaders, donor agencies, the scientific community, and the general public have begun to appreciate the potentially catastrophic consequences of the AIDS epidemic. Without effective, inexpensive, and widely available antiviral therapeutic options, the highest priority is to prevent transmission. Because sexual transmission is responsible for the majority of adult infections, public health education promoting condom use and discouraging multiple sexual partners will have the greatest impact (Fig. 2-4). It is now well documented that sexual practices among homosexual men in the United States and among some groups of prostitutes in Africa have changed dramatically in response to educational programs. The percentage of prostitutes in an impoverished area of Nairobi who reported condom use with some clients rose from 8 percent in 1985 to more than 90 percent by 1987, due in part to an education campaign by the Kenyan Ministry of Health. HIV education programs need to be integrated with programs for STD control, family planning, and maternal and child health at local, national, and international levels. Many countries are implementing two other important strategies, blood-bank screening and sterilization of injection equipment, to reduce HIV transmission. With mounting evidence that certain STDs greatly facilitate sexual transmission of HIV, it is clear that programs to control these diseases must be strengthened, not only to reduce STD-related morbidity and mortality but also to decrease sexual transmission of HIV. The potential for rapid spread of HIV within high-risk populations has been demonstrated in developing countries, as well as in developed countries. In the face of this explosive and deadly pandemic, a coordinated international approach is required if control

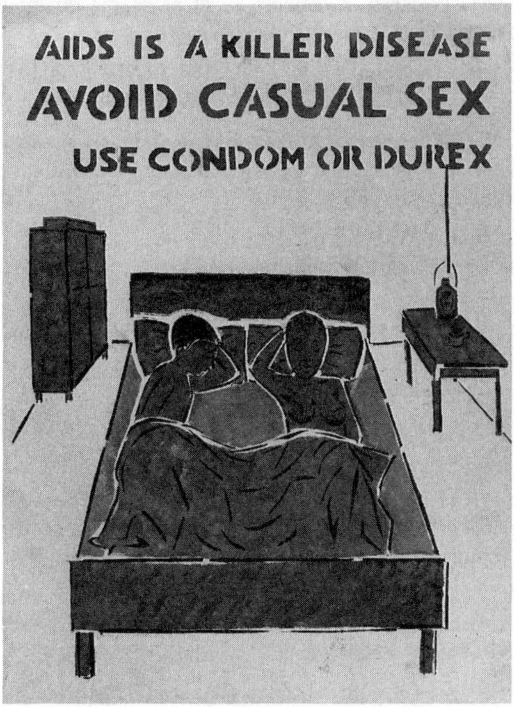

Figure 2-4. This poster is part of an AIDS education program in West Africa.

efforts are to be successful. A Delphi survey showed that a panel of knowledgeable experts believed that up to 50 percent of the estimated 5 million cases of HIV infections projected to occur over the next decade could be prevented by rigorous and coordinated HIV and AIDS prevention programs, using existing technology.[15]

REFERENCES

1. Piot P, Plummer FA, Mhalu FS, et al. AIDS: An international perspective. *Science* 1988;239:573–579.
2. Rwandan HIV Seroprevalence Study Group. Nationwide community-based serological survey of HIV-1 and other human retrovirus infections in a central African country. *Lancet* 1989;1:941–943.
3. Berkley SF, Widy-Wirski R, Okware SI, et al. Risk factors associated with HIV infection in Uganda. *J Infect Dis* 1989;160:22–30.

4. De Cock KM, Porter A, Odehouri K, et al. Rapid emergence of AIDS in Abidjan, Ivory Coast. *Lancet* 1989;2:408–410.

5. Cortes E, Detels R, Aboulafia D, et al. HIV-1, HIV-2, and HTLV-1 infection in high-risk groups in Brazil. *N Engl J Med* 1989;320:955–958.

6. Larson A. Social context of human immunodeficiency virus transmission in Africa: Historical and cultural bases of East and Central African sexual relations. *Rev Infect Dis* 1989;11:716–731.

7. Kreiss JK, Koech D, Plummer FA, et al. AIDS virus infection in Nairobi prostitutes: Spread of the epidemic to East Africa. *N Engl J Med* 1986; 314:414–418.

8. Cameron DW, Simonsen JN, D'Costa LJ, et al. Female to male transmission of human immunodeficiency virus type 1: Risk factors for seroconversion in men. *Lancet* 1989;2:403–407.

9. Quinn TC, Mann JM, Curran JW, et al. AIDS in Africa: An epidemiologic paradigm. *Science* 1986;234:955–963.

10. Greenberg AE, Nguyen-Dinh P, Mann JM, et al. The association between malaria, blood transfusions, and HIV seropositivity in a pediatric population in Kinshasa, Zaire. *JAMA* 1988;259:545–549.

11. Ryder RW, Nsa W, Hassig SE, et al. Perinatal transmission of the human immunodeficiency virus type 1 to infants of seropositive women in Zaire. *N Engl J Med* 1989;320:1637–1642.

12. Quinhoes EP, Koefman S, Noronha CP, et al. Opportunistic infections and neoplasms related to all known cases in the municipality of Rio de Janeiro, Brazil during the period 1982–1987. [Abstract 5065]. *IV International Conference on AIDS*. Stockholm, Sweden, June 1988.

13. Reeves WC, Cueves M, Arosemena J, et al. Human immunodeficiency virus infection in the Republic of Panama. *Am J Trop Med* 1988;39:398–405.

14. Vittecog D, May T, Roue RT, et al. Acquired immunodeficiency syndrome after travelling in Africa: An epidemiological study in seventeen Caucasian patients. *Lancet* 1987;1:612–615.

15. Sato PA, Chin J, Mann JM. Review of AIDS and HIV infection: Global epidemiology and statistics, 1989. AIDS, in press.

3

Public Health Measures to Prevent and Control HIV Infection and AIDS

Robert W. Wood

Public health officials and primary physicians can take steps on three levels to control AIDS. These levels include controlling disease transmission (primary prevention); controlling or delaying disease progression (secondary prevention); and preventing or ameliorating disease complications, including the impact of disease due to HIV on the community (tertiary prevention).

Primary prevention consists mainly of education to reduce risk-taking behaviors. Although no drugs are presently capable of eradicating HIV infection, secondary prevention is becoming increasingly possible. Zidovudine (formerly azidothymidine or AZT) appears to delay progression to overt AIDS and to prolong survival of those with AIDS, but there is no evidence that antiviral therapy alters infectivity or the potential for transmission of HIV. Infected persons should be counseled to avoid behaviors that may transmit HIV or activate HIV-infected lymphocytes, which may enhance HIV replication. Such behaviors include IV drug use and further exposure to STDs through unprotected sexual activity with multiple partners. Primary care providers can monitor immune system status and facilitate early identification and treatment of common infections; prophylactic antibiotics can prevent some opportunistic infections. Tertiary prevention is possible in the social context by reducing unnecessary fear and negative reactions to persons at risk or infected with HIV and in the medical context by developing efficient, comprehensive care systems (Table 3-1).

As the AIDS epidemic continues, it is clear that the resources of public health departments will not be sufficient. The proactive assistance of physicians and other health care providers in AIDS control is crucial, as are expanded resources at federal, state, and local government levels. This chapter is designed to help physicians fulfill their important roles in AIDS

Table 3-1. AIDS control programs in Seattle - King County

Primary Prevention

Education
- At-risk populations
  - Risk reduction via media
  - One-to-one counseling
  - HIV antibody testing
  - Partner notification
  - Extended counseling
  - Information about services
- General community
  - Diminish fear
  - Risk reduction

Secondary Prevention

One-to-one counseling
Clinical services to seropositive individuals
Experimental antiviral chemotherapy

Tertiary Prevention

Community planning, e.g., AIDS task forces
Comprehensive home support
Case management
Fear reduction

control and understand current public health AIDS control programs. Emphasis is on primary prevention; secondary and tertiary control measures are addressed further in Chaps. 11 and 12.

GENERAL APPROACHES TO PRIMARY AIDS PREVENTION

Primary prevention of many communicable diseases is achieved through vaccines; drugs that eradicate the agent(s) in carriers; and sanitary measures, vector elimination, disease screening, and education. Quarantine or other restrictions on the liberty of infected persons may be of assistance in controlling a few diseases.

No vaccines or drugs are presently available to combat the spread of HIV. Because the virus is not spread by casual contact or insect vectors, sanitary measures, vector elimination, and quarantine are not important in preventing AIDS. Thus, education is the cornerstone of HIV control, and screening for HIV infection contributes importantly to educational efforts.

BEHAVIOR CHANGE STRATEGIES

Mass media approaches

Reducing behaviors that place persons at risk for AIDS requires specific knowledge of and attitudes about AIDS that translate into intentions and behaviors. Persons must first know that AIDS is serious and that anyone with substantial exposure can be vulnerable, but also that all persons can reduce their risk of infection. The hope is to motivate all persons to assess their risk for infection, which also requires that they know about its cause (HIV) and transmission. If this self-assessment demonstrates actual (or potential) behavior that could result in HIV infection, individuals need to identify behavioral alternatives that will be acceptable, achievable, and possible to maintain. This requires a realistic appraisal of their own attitudes and of those around them whom they value.[1] Actual risk experience also raises the need to consider HIV antibody testing (see below).

Knowledge about AIDS, its seriousness, cause, and transmission, has been disseminated through news media, including television (apparently the major source of information for both majority and minority populations),[2] newspapers, magazines, and (in 1988) the first-ever federal government mailout focusing on a major health problem. Public health programs, with media assistance, have highlighted three important messages for the general population: AIDS is preventable if people avoid behaviors that transmit HIV; AIDS is not spread by nonintimate casual contact such as occurs in public settings or in the workplace; and compassionate, helpful approaches are essential as more people become afflicted. AIDS is among the leading cause of years of potential life lost (see Chap. 1), and health education should emphasize sexual abstinence prior to marriage, mutual monogamy, and sexual safety (correct use of condoms and lubricants containing nonoxynol-9). In addition, everyone should be taught that drugs and alcohol can cloud judgment about sexual decision making.

Specific community approaches

Specific messages have been aimed at the populations that epidemiology has shown to be at risk: gay men, IV drug users, persons who have received multiple transfusions of blood or blood products, the sexual partners of persons in these groups, minorities, and impoverished persons. Specific information is being provided increasingly to youth because many are sexually active or use drugs before they leave high school. A recent Harris poll indicated that 67 percent of teenagers are sexually active by age 17 and that only 47 percent of males and 25 percent of females report using condoms.

In addition to mass media approaches, successful AIDS information dissemination to at-risk groups has involved programs developed and delivered by local workers and community-based organizations, including information campaigns (Fig. 3-1), small group parties (modeled after Tupperware parties),[3] and community outreach, especially for IV drug users.[4]

According to Fishbein and Ajzen,[5] behaviors result from a summation of attitudinal and normative influences. Attitudes are the feelings that can be identified within an individual that influence such things as preference for sexual partner, sexual object or aim, use of drugs, and avoidance of disease or death. Normative influences come from persons who have the most power in modifying the individual's behavior, including the police, significant family members, and friends. Specific information can significantly modify both attitudinal and normative beliefs. For example, in San Francisco "Stop AIDS" parties are believed to have been successful in reducing risk among gay men because these men gathered within their social groups

Figure 3-1. The Northwest AIDS Foundation and the AIDS Prevention Project (Seattle) target educational materials to gay as well as general audiences.

to discuss the risk of AIDS and to develop a new sense of community sexual norms. Other programs use more formal community approaches, especially within minority groups, to provide specific, acceptable knowledge about AIDS that changes attitudes and norms.[6]

Safer sex and needle hygiene programs

Even before it was known with certainty that AIDS is caused by a virus, the evidence that it was spread sexually suggested that condoms might reduce transmission, and condoms soon became the centerpiece of safer sex campaigns aimed at gay men. Condoms have been handed out in the tens of thousands in everything from matchbook covers (with instructions printed on the inside) to fortune cookies.

Using similar reasoning, in 1987 AIDS control programs in San Francisco and New York began distributing small bottles of bleach (shown to inactivate HIV in contaminated needles) to users of IV drugs. Bottles had instruction labels printed in English and Spanish and were often provided in small kits along with condoms, condom instructions, lubricants, and skin disinfectants. Now such programs are common in nearly all cities with identified users of illicit IV drugs.

In cities in Europe and Australia, and now in the United States, the natural next step—needle-exchange programs—has been undertaken by departments of public health: exchanging used needles for an equal number of sterile ones. Such programs also offer packages of bleach and condoms; staff are available for education, treatment referral, and other forms of assistance. To date, there is no evidence of increasing drug use in these cities, but there is preliminary evidence of a decrease in dirty needles in the streets, parks, and alleyways; of self-reported reductions in needle-sharing and in sexual risk-taking behaviors; and of increasing acceptance of treatment for drug addiction among needle-exchange users.[7]

Individual prevention of HIV infection

In addition to primary prevention strategies aimed at the general population or groups of individuals, a major AIDS control strategy employed by public health workers has been to provide individualized, one-to-one risk screening, HIV risk-reduction counseling, and HIV testing when appropriate. Care providers can play an important role by supplying information about AIDS in their one-to-one patient contacts, especially with persons at risk for HIV infection. Such individualized assessment coupled with education about reducing risk, especially if consistent with public health messages, may have a more profound impact than do mass media approaches in reducing disease spread and fear while demonstrating care and compassion.

One-to-one risk-reduction counseling is especially important for high-risk individuals. Physicians must first learn to recognize these individuals, who do not always fit common stereotypes.[8] Men who have sex with other men are a diverse group that includes husbands, clergy, doctors, and politicians, many of whom may not think of themselves as homosexual or bisexual. Similarly, IV drug users, prostitutes, and other persons at risk are not always easily recognized. Providers often must confront their own beliefs as they delve more deeply into their patients' lifestyles and sexual behaviors. To uncover HIV infection or risk, caregivers must be willing to discuss such issues and render appropriate assistance (see Chap. 12). Strong moralistic feelings are difficult to conceal and may impede gathering data and providing helpful advice.

Testing for HIV infection

The disease prevention value of serologic screening for HIV antibodies is controversial, but anecdotally it may be powerful. Most persons develop measurable antibodies within 3–12 weeks of being infected, and remain permanently infected and contagious thereafter. Most public health authorities believe that voluntary screening, combined with AIDS education, can be helpful in motivating those at risk to adopt safer lifestyles. Some data suggest that both HIV-seronegative and -seropositive persons shift toward safer sexual behavior after testing and counseling.[9] Recent data suggesting that treatment with zidovudine may delay progression to overt AIDS serve as an additional rationale for testing.

Forces that interfere with the motivation of at-risk persons to seek testing and counseling services must be minimized and those that promote the value of these services must be enhanced. Interfering factors include lack of knowledge about the benefits of HIV testing and counseling; fears about coercion and loss of liberty associated with testing; and the beliefs that nothing can be done for the seropositive person or that needed services are not available or affordable. HIV testing in most settings should be voluntary, after at least verbal informed consent, and the records of testing must be protected with careful procedures to maintain confidentiality or anonymity.

Because HIV testing that is mandatory—other than in blood or tissue banks—or without informed consent may contribute to fears of coercion or loss of liberty, these approaches should generally be avoided. Many persons most in need of screening, counseling, and testing appear to be frightened away by fears of governmental lists or infractions of rights, even at the risk of their health. Prior to the current strong arguments for HIV testing based on the benefits of early diagnosis, immune system monitoring, and the use of zidovudine and prophylactic medications, some gay political leaders argued that serologic testing served mostly to subject already stigmatized persons to further discrimination, including loss of insurance, housing, or employment. They argued that everyone, especially those already at risk for infection, should practice only safer sex (see Chap. 12, table 12-1) and that testing should not be needed for AIDS prevention. Similarly, because all persons should be assumed to harbor HIV or other communicable pathogens and should be handled in health care facilities as if infected (see Chap. 14), routine testing was also thought to be unnecessary. Routine hospital testing is still not advocated by most public health authorities.

Testing should be done with the patient's understanding, consent, and only with appropriate counseling; it may be the test-related counseling, rather than the test result itself, which produces the major disease-control effect of screening. Persons likely to have positive test results should be given substantial pretest counseling that covers the medical history, the pros and cons of testing, and resources for dealing with a positive result (see Chap. 6). Care providers should give test results in person, not by telephone or mail, to those at substantial risk of infection. Such personal interaction permits more counseling and allows the caregiver to evaluate the patient's response. Regardless of whether testing is ordered primarily for diagnostic purposes or as a component of risk-reduction counseling, the person ordering the test *must* provide both pre- and posttest counseling or arrange for another qualified professional to do so.

Anonymous counseling and testing services (i.e., without the patient's name or other identifying information) usually should be a local option because, despite the public health department's excellent record in maintaining the confidentiality of such sensitive information, some persons believe that their test results might not remain confidential. The benefit of testing depends on the patient's awareness of the test result more than on the testing agency's or physician's knowledge of the patient's identity. After Oregon made anonymous testing available, there was a substantial increase in the number of persons counseled and in the proportion and number of persons who became aware of their seropositive status.[10]

Some programs designed for one-to-one counseling and testing of higher-risk persons have been overwhelmed by large numbers of frightened but very low-risk persons whose test results are routinely negative and who simply could have been reassured and warned to "play it safe" henceforth. Except to relieve anxiety, counseling and testing usually are not useful for persons with no perceptible risk for HIV exposure. However, media-generated anxiety may be severe, and the psychological benefits of testing these persons may be substantial. In such low-risk situations, it may be appropriate to provide test results by telephone. In addition, in some settings (e.g., in cities with a high incidence of IV drug use–associated HIV infection), the prevalence of HIV infection in apparently low-risk heterosexual adults may be expected to rise.

Lack of access to primary care, therapeutic drugs, and other resources for persons with HIV infection is being seen. As physicians who were initially involved are being overwhelmed by the sick, new physicians are reluctant to become involved, and third-party payors are delaying costly decisions, pending more formal studies. Patients and physicians are often caught in a "catch-22" situation that interferes with decision making. Reluctance by providers to render services to at-risk populations could severely impede disease control at all levels.

EXTENDED COUNSELING

Individuals who cannot easily change to low-risk behaviors may need extended counseling. Investigators are exploring how sexual behaviors can be considered and treated as addictions, such as cigarette smoking and alcoholism. Despite evidence of substantial change in the behaviors of gay men, some continue to take risks despite knowledge of the possible consequences. For example, as of 1986, about 10 percent of gay men in San Francisco continued to engage in unprotected receptive anal intercourse. Depression may be an important factor in such cases, and caregivers should be alert to signs of suicidal intent. One approach may be through extended one-to-one or group counseling.

A preliminary survey in Seattle showed that 70 percent of such men and women desire counseling to change this pattern[11] and that some are willing to engage in group or individual counseling. Early studies demonstrate that relapse prevention–model counseling[12] may be successful for some of these persons.

Persons who use illicit IV drugs have also reported substantially reducing their risk-taking behaviors, although not to the same degree as have most gay men.[13] They also seek treatment for their drug addictions more willingly. Those who continue using drugs report concern about AIDS, reduction in needle sharing, and increasing use of substances such as bleach to sterilize needles between uses. IV drug users spread HIV not only by sharing needles, but as often by unprotected sex. Unfortunately, they report less protection against transmission by sex than by needle use.

Because of the intensity of the addictions caused by most illicit injected drugs, "just saying no" is rarely effective. Users need ongoing, long-term treatment—either in the form of substitution, such as with methadone—or through withdrawal accompanied by psychological and social support programs. In most areas of the country, despite recent proposed increases, there is far too little drug treatment capacity to handle the demand, especially for those with few or no financial resources.

PARTNER NOTIFICATION

Partner notification is used routinely to control transmission of gonorrhea and syphilis and is being increasingly applied to HIV infection. There is a general consensus that steps should be taken to ensure that all sexual or needle-sharing partners of HIV-infected persons are notified and that the infected person usually is in the best position to notify his or her partners. There is disagreement as to how vigorously the physician, testing agency, or local health department should pursue partner notification if the index patient is unable or unwilling to do so.

In Washington state, vigorous efforts are made to notify all partners who are believed to be *unsuspecting* of their exposure or risk status—for example, the female sexual partner who is unaware that her partner is bisexual or the partners of IV drug users. State law protects health care providers from criminal charges of breach of the index patient's privacy in notifying unsuspecting partners. In some jurisdictions, health authorities attempt to contact all partners, whether unsuspecting or not, in the belief that personal counseling, confrontation with the fact of HIV exposure, and voluntary HIV antibody testing will induce many of them to adopt safer behaviors. Recent data suggest that these premises are correct for many high-risk group members.[14] In addition, increasing evidence that zidovudine and antibiotic prophylaxis for opportunistic infections can prevent or delay serious morbidity in some HIV-infected persons (see Chap. 11) further supports the rationale for routine partner notification.

Practitioners should counsel infected persons to inform their sexual or needle-sharing partners about AIDS and to encourage them to seek counseling and antibody testing. Practitioners should also know that local public health departments can be consulted for advice about partner notification and that most departments have established protocols, staff, and funding to carry out partner notification. Because these persons have more expertise and time to perform these investigations, they should at least be consulted; in most situations, private providers are encouraged to turn the job over to them.

REPORTING HIV INFECTIONS TO HEALTH AUTHORITIES

In all U.S. states and territories, AIDS cases must be reported to local public health authorities, with identifying information. Some states, such as Washington, also require reporting of persons who have serious HIV-related diseases (CDC Class IV Disease)[15]; as of August 1989, 18 states require reporting of the names of all HIV-infected persons. Ten more states require the reporting of seropositive cases without identifying information.

Reporting the identities of infected persons is controversial. Although it has been argued that reporting permits estimation of the incidence and prevalence of HIV infection to aid in control measures and to plan for future resources, randomized, unlinked serologic surveys probably are more effective for this purpose. Reporting also may assist in partner notification (although the identity of the index seropositive patient is not needed for notification) and help ensure that infected persons can be notified of new developments in health care. However, there is evidence that such reporting, by fostering fears of discrimination or prejudice, can reduce the number of risk-group members who seek testing and counseling and thereby adversely affect HIV control. Physicians should know and adhere to the reporting laws and regulations in their jurisdictions. Even where reporting is required, anonymous HIV testing and counseling services, as discussed, have played an important role and should be retained.

EVIDENCE OF SUCCESS

Programs for disease control appear to be working. McKusick and others[16] have shown substantial changes in the behaviors of gay men, and DesJarlais and Friedman[13] have shown a 50 percent reducton in reported needle sharing and an increased desire for drug treatment among IV drug users in New York City. The incidence of new HIV infection in gay men in San Francisco decreased from an estimated 20–30 percent annually to less than 1 percent annually from 1982 to 1986.[17] Additionally, data from many metropolitan areas in this country and abroad have shown changes in the frequencies of certain STDs including 80–90 percent reductions of rectal gonorrhea, hepatitis, herpes, and syphilis among gay men. In Seattle, the combined total of gonorrhea cases in gay men in public clinics and reported cases of rectal gonorrhea in males decreased from more than 1100 in 1982 to 35 in 1988 (–96 percent). Among some heterosexual populations (notably inner-city drug users and their partners), the incidence of this disease is stable or rising. This pattern indicates the need for more education.

SUMMARY

To control AIDS and minimize its impact, health care practitioners must understand and cooperate with public health strategies. Because of the long interval from HIV infection to overt AIDS, much time already has been lost, and the effects of today's efforts will take years to materialize. Care providers should be actively involved in primary, secondary, and tertiary disease control. All must assist in the education effort because practically all will care for persons with AIDS and HIV infections in the years to come. Innovative approaches now being developed for the care of patients with AIDS will benefit persons with many other chronic diseases by increasing the general quality, accessibility, efficiency, and compassion of the health care system.

REFERENCES

1. Coates TJ, Stall RD, Catania JA, Kegeles SM. Behavioral factors in the spread of HIV infection. *AIDS* 1988;2(suppl 1):S239–S246.
2. Hardy AM, Dawson DA. AIDS knowledge and attitudes for October and November 1988. National Center for Health Statistics: Advance data. April 19, 1989;No.167.
3. AIDS Action Committee. SafetyNet Program: Small group parties for safer sex education. *Am J Public Health* 1989;79:1305.
4. Froner G, Rowniak S. The health outreach team: Taking AIDS education and health care to the streets. *AIDS Education and Prevention* 1989;1(2):105–118.
5. Fishbein M, Ajzen I. *Understanding attitudes and predicting social behavior*. Englewood Cliffs, NJ: Prentice-Hall, 1980.
6. McAllister A, Perry CL, Killer J, et al. Pilot study of smoking, alcohol, and drug abuse prevention. *Am J Public Health* 1980;70:719–721.
7. Stimson GV. Editorial review: Syringe exchange programmes for injecting drug users. *AIDS* 1989;3:253–260.
8. Owen WF. 1980. The clinical approach to the homosexual patient. *Ann Int Med* 93:90–92.
9. Cates W, Handsfield HH. HIV counseling and testing: Does it work? *Am J Public Health* 1988;78:1533–1534.
10. Fehrs LJ, Foster LR, Fox V, et al. Trial of anonymous versus confidential human immunodeficiency virus testing. *Lancet* 1988;2:379–381.
11. Roffman RA, Gillmore MR, Gilchrist LD, et al. Continuing unsafe sex: Assessing need for AIDS-prevention counseling. *Public Health Rep*, in press.
12. Marlatt GA, Gordon JR, eds. *Relapse prevention*. New York: Guilford Press, 1985.
13. DesJarlais DC, Friedman SR. Editorial review: HIV infection among intravenous drug users: Epidemiology and risk reduction. *AIDS* 1987;1:67–76.
14. Jones JL, Wykoff RF, Gamble WB, et al. Partner acceptability of health department notification of HIV exposure, South Carolina. Fifth International Conference on AIDS, Montreal, June 4–9, 1989.
15. Centers for Disease Control. Classification system for human T lymphotropic

virus, type III/lymphadenopathy associated virus infections. *MMWR* 1986;35:334–338.

16. McKusick L, Wiley JA, Coates TJ, et al. Reported changes in the sexual behavior of men at risk for AIDS, San Francisco, 1982–1984: The AIDS behavioral research project. *Public Health Rep* 1985;100:622–629.
17. Bacchetti P, Moss, AR. Incubation period of AIDS in San Francisco. *Nature* 1989;338:251–253.

4

HIVs and Related Simian Retroviruses

Robert W. Coombs
Michael G. Katze

Retroviruses have been implicated as important animal pathogens for more than 60 years. However, they were identified as etiologic agents in human disease only in the past decade. In this chapter, we review the biology of human retroviruses and describe in particular the pathophysiology of HIV infection.

RETROVIRUS DEFINITION AND CLASSIFICATION

The family Retroviridiae is a large group of ubiquitous viruses that infect all classes of vertebrates. Retroviruses are named for a unique, viral-encoded enzyme called *reverse transcriptase*. In a reverse of the normal flow of information from DNA to RNA, reverse transcriptase makes a DNA copy of the single-stranded viral RNA genome, hence the prefix *retro*. Retroviruses are characterized morphologically by their electron microscopic appearance and by their genomic, antigenic, and physiopathologic characteristics.

Although many retroviruses can cause cytopathology in their host cells, most replicate without killing the infected cell. A persistent infection may result, or the infected cell may be transformed and a malignancy induced. Based on these characteristics, human retroviruses are divided into two subfamilies: the transforming oncoviruses (Oncovirinae) and the cytopathic lentiviruses (Lentivirinae).

While differing in both morphology and physiopathology, these two human retrovirus groups share the following characteristics:

They bud from the cell surface.

They have an external envelope containing a large molecular weight, external receptor glycoprotein, and a smaller, anchoring, transmembrane glycoprotein.

They possess a high molecular weight, single-stranded RNA genome.

They have internal structural proteins that surround the RNA genome.

They encode an RNA-dependent DNA polymerase (reverse transcriptase).

Retroviruses replicate by a double-stranded DNA intermediate known as a *provirus*. Proviral DNA often integrates into the host cell's genome but may also take an extrachromosomal, circular form. In addition to reverse transcriptase, at least two host cell polymerases are required: a DNA-dependent DNA polymerase for making multiple copies of the intermediate proviral DNA and an RNA polymerase II for transcribing the retrovirus proviral DNA into messenger RNA (mRNA). The general scheme for human retroviral replication is shown in Fig. 4-1.

ONCOVIRUSES

Oncoviruses cause many animal malignancies and characteristically may immortalize cells in vitro. In humans the prototype oncoviruses are the human T-cell lymphotropic viruses (HTLV) type I and type II. HTLV-I causes adult T-cell leukemia and may be linked to the degenerative central nervous system disease tropical spastic paraparesis. HTLV-II has been isolated from some patients with hairy cell leukemia. The HTLV-I virus has CD4+ cell tropism that results in both a direct in vitro cytopathic effect (syncytium formation with multinucleated giant cells) and an uncontrolled proliferation, causing leukemia in vivo, with subsequent immunosuppression and susceptibility to opportunistic infection. These events may occur after decades of latency if the infection was acquired early in childhood or after only a few years if the infection was acquired in adulthood.

Recently, serologic surveys to detect HTLV-I and -II infection have been developed. At present these assays do not distinguish between the two types. Overall, the prevalence of HTLV-I and -II in the general population of the United States is low (<1 percent). However, in a study of IV drug users in Queens, New York, the prevalence of serum antibodies to HTLV-I and -II was 9 percent and 18 percent, respectively. Dual infection with HTLV-I or -II and with HIV was found in 27 percent of black IV drug users from the same area. The impact of this "double jeopardy" on the expression of either HTLV- or HIV-induced disease is unknown but worrisome, as HTLV-I

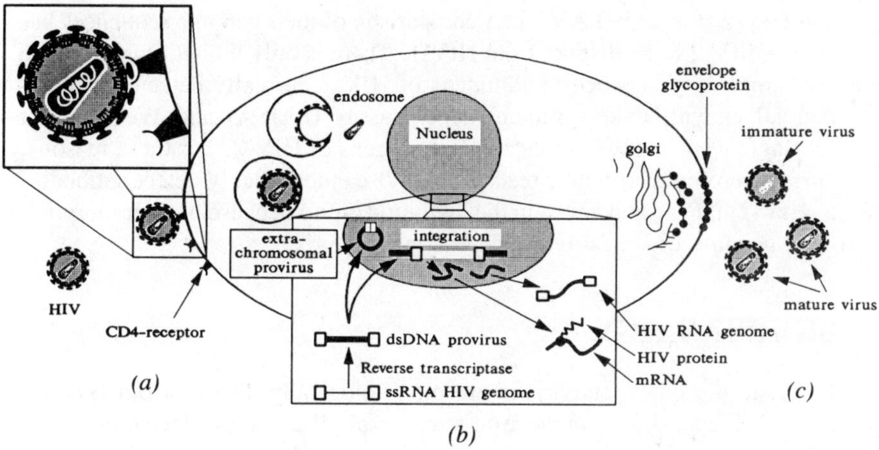

Figure 4.1. HIV replication cycle. (*a*) Attachment and penetration. The virus attaches to the CD4 receptor by the viral gp120 *env* protein and enters the cell by endocytosis. Fusion of the viral envelope with the endosome releases the viral core that contains the single-stranded RNA genome and reverse transcriptase enzyme. (*b*) Replication. The reverse transcriptase makes a DNA copy of the RNA genome, and the resulting double-stranded DNA provirus either integrates into the host genome or remains extrachromosomal. Transcription of the HIV DNA copy into mRNA is then followed by translation of mRNA to viral protein. Several accessory control genes are responsible for regulating viral expression at this stage. (*c*) Assembly. The viral *env* glycoprotein incorporates into the host-cell membrane and serves as a condensation site for the nucleocapsid. The viral particles then bud from the cell surface, and the viral core undergoes further extracellular condensation to form the morphologically mature virion.

infection increases HIV-1 gene expression. Thus, dually infected persons may have a substantially greater likelihood of rapidly developing AIDS or human T-cell leukemia.

LENTIVIRUSES

The lentivirus subfamily of retroviruses causes slowly progressive diseases with lymphotropic and neurotropic features in both humans and ungulates (horses, sheep, cattle, and goats). These viruses can produce cytopathology in their target cells, including syncytium formation in vitro. The only known members of the human lentivirus group belong to the human immunodeficiency viruses, the etiologic agents of AIDS. These viruses have a tropism for CD4+ T cells and other cells with the CD4 receptor. The HIV group is more diverse than was previously thought. Two distinct subtypes of HIV have been defined: HIV-1 (formerly HTLV-III, LAV-1, and ARV);

and HIV-2 (formerly LAV-2). A comparison of their genome sequences has shown HIV-2 to be distinct from HIV-1. There is only limited immunologic cross-reactivity between the antigens of HIV-1 currently detected in commercial enzyme-linked immunosorbent assay (ELISA) and Western blot serologic tests and the corresponding antigens of HIV-2. For these reasons, current serologic screening tests for HIV-1 cannot reliably detect antibodies to HIV-2. HIV-1 and -2 are in the lentivirus group because of their morphology, genome organization, and protein structure.

MORPHOLOGY

HIV and the other lentiviruses are morphologically distinct from HTLV-I and -II. Figure 4-2 is an electron micrograph of an HIV-infected cell. The electron microscopic appearance of this virus is characterized by a conical, electron-dense center. All the retroviruses have a glycoprotein-studded envelope and are approximately 100 nm in size. The conical nucleocapsid core contains the single-stranded RNA genome, structural proteins, and reverse transcriptase.

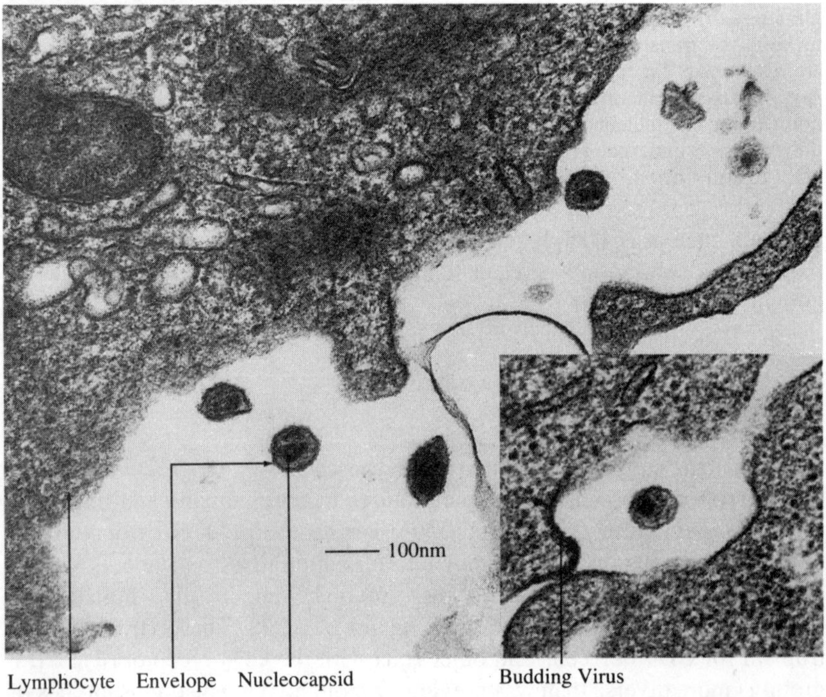

Figure 4-2. An electron micrograph of a lymphocyte infected with HIV.

GENOME ORGANIZATION AND PROTEIN STRUCTURE

The genes of HIV and the proteins they encode are important in pathogenesis, are the potential targets for new antiviral drugs, and are of great importance in understanding the current basis for serologic diagnosis and recent developments in vaccine research. The genes coding for the major structural (i.e., nonregulatory) proteins of HIV are arranged in the left-to-right (5' → 3') direction and are designated *gag, pol,* and *env* (Fig. 4-3). These genes are flanked by the regulatory-integration sequences in the duplicated long terminal repeat segments. In addition, four accessory genes regulate viral expression and infectivity, although the process is not yet understood.

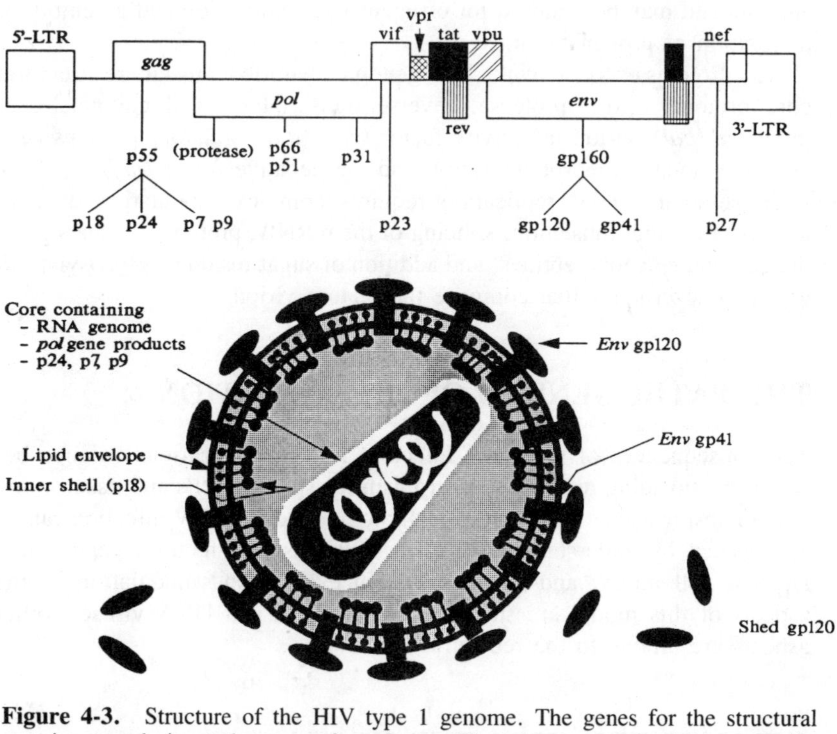

Figure 4-3. Structure of the HIV type 1 genome. The genes for the structural proteins are designated *gag, pol,* and *env*. The accessory genes necessary for controlling viral replication and infectivity are *vif, tat, rev,* and *nef*. An eighth gene, *vpr,* and a ninth gene, *vpu,* have currently unknown functions. The duplicate long terminal repeats contain recognition sequences required for integration into the host-cell genome, an inducible host-cell transcription factor, and the regulatory *tat* protein. The major translational products and their locations in the mature virion also are shown.

One of these accessory genes, designated *negative factor (nef)*, apparently has a negative effect on HIV replication and may help to keep HIV latent. The other three accessory genes are necessary for viral production and infectivity. The *transactivator (tat)* gene is a split gene flanking the *env* gene. (Note: A gene product is said to act in trans when it regulates another gene.) This gene product up-regulates both HIV transcription and translation and can be considered autostimulatory. Another accessory split gene flanking the *env* gene is the *regulator of expression of virion proteins (rev)*. This gene product has a different regulatory effect and enables the integrated virus to produce selectively either regulatory proteins or virion components. The fourth accessory gene, *virion infectivity factor (vif),* is apparently necessary for the normal infectivity of HIV, although how it does this is unknown. An eighth gene, *viral protein R (vpr)*, has an unknown function. Recently, a ninth gene, *viral protein U (vpu),* has been located between *tat* and *env* and may be required for efficient viral replication and assembly or maturation of progeny virions.

The proteins encoded by the HIV genome identified thus far are structural core proteins *(gag);* protease, reverse transcriptase, and endonuclease-integrase *(pol)*; virion infectivity factor *(vif)*; transregulatory proteins *(tat, rev)*; envelope glycoproteins *(env)*; and the negative factor *(nef)*.

In summary, HIV replication requires complex modulation of both transcription and translation, splicing of the mRNA, proteolytic cleavage of the *gag* and *env* polypeptides, and addition of sugar residues (glycosylation) to form the proteins that compose the mature virion.

THE PATHOGENESIS OF HIV INFECTION

The consequences of retroviral infection reflect a precarious balance between the invading retrovirus, its tropism for specific cells and tissues, and human host resistance. The physiopathologic model of HIV infection can be approached by understanding viral mechanisms of infection, persistence, latency, cell injury, and immune system evasion and modulation. Some aspects of this model are shared by other RNA and DNA viruses; other aspects are unique to the retrovirus group.

VIRAL ENTRY INTO THE HOST

HIV transmission requires either parenteral or intimate mucous membrane exposure to the virus. Transmission by fomites is unlikely because HIV, as an enveloped virus, is sensitive to several envelope-disruptive forces of the environment, such as high temperature, surface tension (e.g., drying), and detergents. The concentration of virus in body fluids to which a person is exposed—for example, the small number of infectious HIV particles in saliva versus the large number in blood—is an important determinant of transmission. Secretory IgA from the infected host may restrict HIV salivary transmission, as 70 percent of AIDS patients have salivary IgA against the *env* proteins. The precise mechanisms of transmission are not yet well understood, and an animal model system is needed for further study.

TARGET-CELL TROPISM AND VIRUS-RECEPTOR INTERACTIONS

Susceptible cells are required for the process of adsorption, penetration, and uncoating. For HIV, the CD4 antigen (i.e., T4 or related antigen) is the specific virus receptor. This receptor is a 62-kDa glycoprotein that characterizes the CD4 helper-inducer lymphocyte subset. The HIV gp120 *env* binds specifically to the CD4 receptor. HIV infection is associated with a complete loss of CD4 antigen on infected T cells, and their ultimate death results in a decreased T4:T8 ratio.

The CD4 T cell is not the only cell type infected by HIV. Other cells, such as the monocyte-macrophage, express the CD4+ antigen, especially when activated. HIV infection of monocytes and macrophages does not invariably lead to cell lysis and death, as in the T4 lymphocytes. Monocyte-macrophages infected with HIV disseminate HIV to target organs and serve as a reservoir for virus persistence, a feature shared with some other lentiviruses. Other cells permissive and semipermissive for HIV infection include B lymphocytes positive for Epstein-Barr virus, endothelial cells from established Kaposi's sarcoma, promyelocytes and proerythrocytes, Langerhans' cells of the skin, follicular dendritic cells, and several others, some of which do not express the CD4 antigen. Brain infection with HIV appears to be associated with a mononuclear inflammatory infiltrate, although some evidence exists for infection of primary central nervous system cells that may express a CD4-related antigen. Thus, the number of infected cells expressing HIV gene products in the body is large, and the cell types are diverse.

GENOMIC DIVERSITY

Within the *env* gene, localized regions of extraordinary hypervariability are interspersed with well-conserved (nonvariable) regions. One well-conserved region of the envelope encodes the CD4 attachment site. The degree of variability in the envelope gene is unique to the lentiviruses. The variation may be due to errors in reverse transcription, leading to substitutions and misreading. The mutation rate in the *env* gene is 1 million times greater than that of DNA viruses and 10 to 100 times greater than that of other retroviruses. This extraordinary hypervariability corresponds to amino acid changes of as much as 20 percent among divergent HIV-1 isolates. These regions of hypervariability may modify several biologic properties, including tissue tropism, virulence, replication rate, and sensitivity to antiviral chemotherapy, and may allow the virus to evade the immune response. It is apparent, however, that even in an individual person, several different strains of HIV-1 can be identified.

LATENCY AND PERSISTENCE

For any viral infection to persist, viral gene expression must be restricted. Three patterns of restricted expression are known:

Latent infection, characterized by intermittent episodes of acute disease with no virus detected between episodes (e.g., oral-labial or genital herpes simplex virus).

Chronic infection, in which the virus is always demonstrable but disease is absent (e.g., cytomegalovirus).

Persistent infections, characterized by a long incubation period with slowly increasing amounts of transcriptional-translational products and, eventually, symptomatic disease (e.g., subacute sclerosing panencephalitis from measles virus infection).

The lentiviruses, HIV in particular, share features from all three patterns but are best described as persistent infections. The HIV provirus integrates randomly in the infected host-cell genome, but most proviral DNA remains extrachromosomal. The degree of viral transcription and translation depends on the infected CD4+ cell's stage of differentiation. That stage, in turn, is probably related to exogenous antigen stimulation, that is, exogenous antigen stimulation may promote HIV-1 replication. Integration of human retroviruses differs from that of certain other animal retroviruses in that no transforming genes (oncogenes) are associated with the viral genome, and the proviral genome is not regularly inserted next to a host-transforming gene. Proviral integration is not only important in defining the pathologic mechanisms of the retrovirus group per se, but it also suggests that current chemotherapeutic interventions directed against actively replicating virus will not "cure" cells latently infected with HIV proviral DNA.

MECHANISMS OF CYTOPATHOLOGY

A dilemma in understanding HIV physiopathology is the mechanism by which the CD4+ T-cell population is depleted. It appears that HIV-1 can cause CD4 cell depletion by both direct (cytopathic) and indirect mechanisms. Current studies suggest that one can detect HIV-1 DNA in bone marrow and peripheral blood mononuclear cells in only about 1:100 to 1:10,000 CD4+ cells. However, HIV-1–infected cells expressing gp120 may fuse with uninfected CD4 cells, causing syncytium formation and leaving these fused cells dysfunctional. Similarly, HIV-1 envelope glycoprotein is shed from infected cells. This glycoprotein may bind to CD4 receptors, be internalized and processed, and render this cell susceptible to autoimmune cytolysis by the patient's own CD8+ cells. The CD4 antigen, in addition to being the HIV receptor, directly participates in vitro in cell fusion between infected and uninfected CD4+ cell lines. Introducing HIV envelope glycoprotein into the infected cell membrane destabilizes the membrane and probably causes cytoskeletal alterations in the microtubules, microfilaments, and intermediate filaments that are required for syncytium formation and for viral assembly, budding, and release. The cytopathic feature of HIV appears to reside in the carboxy terminus of the transmembrane glycoprotein gp41. It thus appears that infection in one CD4 cell causes agglutination and fusion of other uninfected cells, leading to their subsequent dysfunction and destruction.

As shown in Fig. 4-4, the major feature of this model is that HIV replication may be promoted by repeated rounds of antigenic stimulation in vivo (e.g., by concurrent infection with other viruses, bacteria, fungi, and protozoans, and by exposure to allogenic cells such as are found in semen and blood).

Successive cycles of HIV latency and expression result from fine tuning of the regulatory *tat, rev,* and *nef* genes. In turn, *env* and *gag* mRNAs accumulate, followed by a burst of viral replication, leading to cell death with depletion of the CD4+ T-cell population and subsequent immunosuppression.

IMMUNOPATHOGENESIS

As mentioned, lymphotropic infection by human and lower primate retroviruses characteristically results in immunosuppression. In the case of HIV infection, selective failure of both adaptive immunity (depletion of the CD4+ helper-inducer subset of lymphocytes) and natural immunity (large granular lymphocytes) results in the immune imbalance. Such imbalance

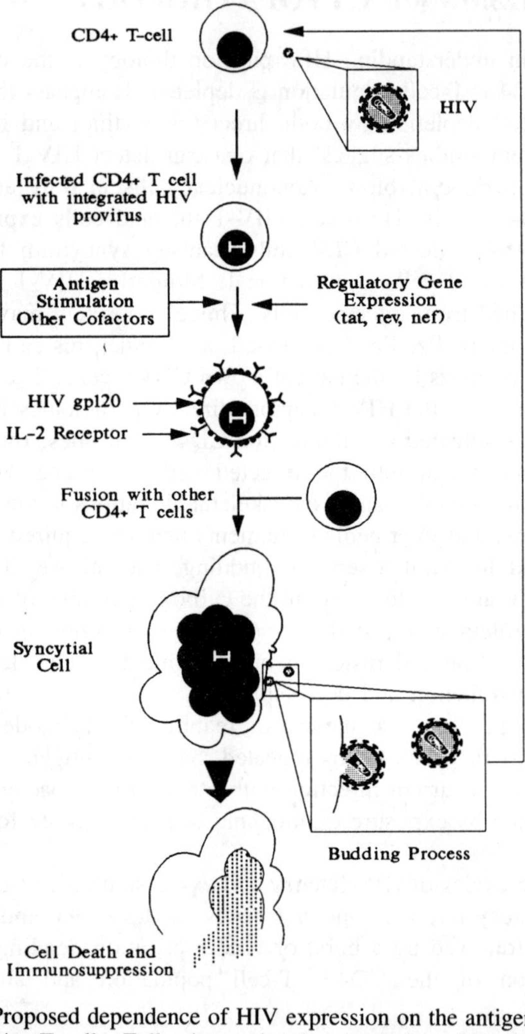

Figure 4-4. Proposed dependence of HIV expression on the antigenic stimulation of infected CD4+ T cells. Following antigenic stimulation of the latently infected CD4+ T cell, HIV is expressed through complex and incompletely understood mechanisms involving the *tat, rev,* and *nef* regulatory genes. Infected cells expressing viral envelope glycoprotein (gp120) and IL-2 receptors fuse with uninfected CD4+ cells, form syncytia, express virus, and then die in an accelerated fashion. This eventually produces an immunodeficiency that usually progresses to AIDS. In the absence of suitable antigenic stimulation, HIV probably remains either latent in the infected CD4+ T cell or at a very low level of persistent expression. (Adapted from Zagury D, Bernard J, Leonard R, et al. Long-term cultures of HTLV-III–infected T cells: A model of cytopathology of T-cell depletion in AIDS. *Science* 1986;231:850–853.)

leaves the patient susceptible to opportunistic infections and malignancies. The CD4+ lymphocyte population normally represents approximately 60 percent of T cells and contains effectors for delayed hypersensitivity, as well as inducers for killer T-cell generation, B-cell differentiation into immunoglobulin-secreting plasma cells, and active suppressor-cell development. This contrasts to the CD8+ population, which is not infected by HIV. The CD8+ subset normally represents approximately 30 percent of the T cells and contains effectors for killer T cells and other cells that suppress cell-mediated reactivities and immunoglobulin production.

The functional T-cell defects produced by HIV infection result in decreased lymphokines [interleukin-2, (IL-2)] and decreased helper-inducer functions for other T and B cells, while the defect in the large granular lymphocytes results in decreased alpha-interferon production. In vitro, the CD8+ T cell suppresses viral expression by infected CD4+ T cells. The B-lymphocyte defects result in a decreased antibody response to soluble antigens with concomitant polyclonal elevation of serum immunoglobulins, primarily of the IgG and IgA classes; this stimulation may represent a complex set of interactions involving HIV itself, Epstein-Barr virus, cytomegalovirus, or possibly the newly recognized human herpesvirus type 6. The monocyte defects may result in the spontaneous increase in IL-1 secretion (hence the observed fever with this disease) and possibly in tumor necrosis factor (hence the wasting component of AIDS, although this may be much more complex, with superimposed gastrointestinal infections and malabsorption). A direct immunosuppresive role for HIV *env* or *gag* proteins has not been demonstrated.

A perplexing feature of HIV infection is that the virus persists in lymphocytes and plasma despite antibody production. Neutralizing antibody binds to the HIV envelope gp120 protein and is found in most patients with AIDS and AIDS-related complex (ARC). Although these antibodies reportedly block attachment of the virus in vitro, it is not known whether this confers immunity in vivo. Escape from antibody neutralization may reflect direct cell-to-cell transmission of the virus, a changing antigen expression of the envelope glycoprotein due to hypervariability in the *env* gene, or both. Several investigators have noted that some patients have antibodies that enhance infection of macrophages in vitro.

The pathophysiology of HIV-1 infection of the central nervous system is also unclear. Acute HIV infection can cause aseptic meningitis. More commonly, chronic infection will cause diffuse gray matter disease and result in clinical dementia. Some investigators have suggested that the envelope protein may cause cytokine release, which may be related to some of the cognitive defects found in HIV-infected individuals. Further studies are needed to elucidate this intriguing aspect of HIV pathogenesis.

SIMIAN RETROVIRUSES

Historically, animal models have proved invaluable in studying the pathogenesis of human viral diseases. Studies using nonhuman primates often have paved the way for life-saving vaccines, with poliovirus being the classic example. Chimpanzees are the only animals susceptible to HIV infection; however, infected chimpanzees show no clinical symptoms of an immunosuppressive disease, and not enough chimpanzees are available for the necessary studies. However, nonhuman primates can be infected with simian immunodeficiency virus (SIV), an agent closely related to HIV-2. This agent causes an AIDS-like disease in nonhuman primates. In addition, the simian acquired immunodeficiency virus type-D (SAIDS-D) offers a worthwhile model for pursuing some aspects of HIV pathogenesis.

Simian acquired immunodefiency virus type-D

The SAIDS-D virus is associated with an acquired immunodeficiency syndrome in various macaques that is similar in certain respects to human AIDS. A novel type-D retrovirus, distinct from previously mentioned viruses (human retroviruses are type C), was isolated by cocultivating explants of fibromatous tissue obtained from naturally infected rhesus monkeys *(Macaca mulatta)*. Infected monkeys show an immunodeficiency syndrome characterized by persistent diarrhea, progressive weight loss, anemia, lymphocytopenia, unusual chronic infections, and a peculiar fibromatous tumor called *retroperitoneal fibromatosis*. Immunohistochemical studies have shown factor VIII–related antigen in endothelial and fibroblast-like cells throughout the retroperitoneal fibromatosis lesions similar to that described for Kaposi's sarcoma. Thus, in its progressive form, SAIDS-D causes lymphoid depletion, opportunistic infections, and an unusual neoplasm (retroperitoneal fibromatosis). No cross-reactivity has been found between SAIDS-D virus and the human lentiviruses at either the protein or the nucleic acid level.

Simian immunodeficiency virus

Several primate centers have isolated lentiviruses from macaques *(Macaca nemestrina)*. This simian lentivirus, SIV, is partially related to the human lentiviruses HIV-1 and HIV-2 isolated from patients with AIDS. Serologic analyses reveal that antisera from sick macaques react strongly with HIV core proteins but only weakly with the envelope glycoproteins. Conversely, antisera from HIV-seropositive patients with AIDS show cross-reactivity with SIV core antigens. The in vitro growth characteristics of SIV also are similar to those of HIV. SIV is tropic for CD4+ T cells, and its infectivity can be blocked by CD4 antibodies.

When healthy rhesus monkeys were infected with SIV experimentally, an AIDS-like immunosuppressive disease was induced which often led to death. The animals developed diarrhea and lost as much as 60 percent of their body weight. The absolute number of CD4+ T cells in their peripheral blood lymphocytes decreased to one-half normal as early as 2 weeks following infection. Because the number of circulating CD8+ T cells remained unchanged, the CD4:CD8 ratio decreased. Over time, there was a reduction in the number of both CD4 and CD8 cells and a large increase in the percentage of B cells, similar to that which occurs in HIV infection in humans. Most SIV-infected monkeys will develop an immunodeficiency-like disease and die with a wasting syndrome and of opportunistic infections similar to the pattern in HIV-1 infection in humans. Thus, SIV provides an excellent model analogous to retroviral infections in humans. Major studies of natural and experimental transmission of SIV, SIV vaccines, and testing of antiviral drugs to block SIV infection are underway.

SUMMARY

There are two major subfamilies of retroviruses that infect humans: oncoviruses, represented by HTLV-I and -II, and lentiviruses, represented by the HIV group. Lentiviruses are characterized by their ability to infect and kill the CD4+ lymphocyte; the decrease in CD4+ lymphocytes inverts the CD4+:CD8+ lymphocyte ratio and causes an immune imbalance that leads to the opportunistic infections and malignancies characteristic of AIDS. The progression of this persistent viral infection may depend on the antigenic stimulation and subsequent differentiation of the infected CD4+ cell.

CD4+ cell depletion cannot be attributed to HIV infection of every CD4+ cell; rather, it likely arises from a combination of viral replication, cell fusion between infected and uninfected CD4+ cells, and autoimmune destruction of CD4+ cells triggered by the interaction of shed viral glycoprotein with the CD4+ receptor on uninfected cells.

Hypervariability in the HIV *env* gene probably confers corresponding antigenic variability in envelope glycoproteins. The conseqences of this hypervariability could be due to development of strains resistant to new chemotherapeutic agents or to the immune response produced by natural infection or by candidate vaccines. An animal model of SIV may help to elucidate the physiopathologic mechanisms of HIV infection in humans and facilitate the development of effective drugs and vaccines.

ADDITIONAL READING

Adams SW. Simian T lymphotropic viruses. *Lab Animal* 1987;16:33–39.

Gallo RC. The AIDS retrovirus. *Sci Amer* 1987;256:47–56.

Gallo RC. The first human retrovirus. *Sci Amer* 1986;255:88–98.

Gallo RC, Wong-Staal F. A human T lymphotropic retrovirus (HTLV-III) as the cause of the aquired immunodeficiency syndrome. *Ann Intern Med* 1985;103:679–689.

Haase AT. Pathogenesis of lentivirus infections. *Nature* 1986;322:130–136.

Haseltine WA. Replication and pathogenesis of the AIDS virus. *J Acquired Immune Deficiency Syndromes* 1988;1:217–240.

Haseltine WA, Wong-Staal F. The molecular biology of the AIDS virus. *Sci Amer* 188;259:52–62.

Levy JA. Mysteries of HIV: Challenges for therapy and prevention. *Nature* 1988;339:519–522.

Weiss A, Hollander H, Stobo J. 1985. Acquired immunodeficiency syndrome: Epidemiology, virology, and immunology. *Ann Rev Med* 1985;36:545–562.

Zagury D, Bernard J, Leonard R, et al. Long-term cultures of HTLV-III-infected T cells: A model of cytopathology of T cell depletion in AIDS. *Science* 1986;231:850–853.

5

Laboratory Diagnosis of HIV Infection

Robert W. Coombs
Lynn Goldstein

Persons infected with HIV are usually identified by the presence of antibodies reactive with the retrovirus. With recently developed techniques, HIV can be isolated from nearly all HIV-seropositive individuals. It is fairly easy to develop a clinical suspicion of AIDS given the appropriate signs and symptoms, such as prolonged fever, fatigue or weight loss, onset of opportunistic infections, and a history of membership in a high-risk group for HIV infection: a homosexual or bisexual male, an IV drug user, a recipient of multiple blood-product transfusions, a person having heterosexual contact with a high-risk or HIV-seropositive partner, a native of certain areas of Africa or Haiti, a male or female prostitute, or a child born to parents who are members of these groups. Physicians face a major challenge in diagnosing HIV infection in a person who is asymptomatic, who has atypical signs and symptoms, or who denies being in a high-risk group.

Current clinical and laboratory approaches to the diagnosis of HIV infection are outlined in Table 5-1. For descriptive and technical purposes, laboratory detection of HIV infection can be stratified into assays identifying HIV antibodies; those identifying HIV virus, antigen, or gene products; and indirect markers of HIV infection.

HIV ANTIBODY ASSAYS

Enzyme immunoassays

Enzyme immunoassays were first developed to detect HIV antibodies in infected potential blood donors. These tests have now been adopted for

Table 5-1. Detection of human immunodeficiency virus infection

Clinical Signs and Symptoms of HIV Infection

Not sensitive, as most initial infections are asymptomatic

Opportunistic infections are highly specific indicators for HIV infection when other recognized causes of immunodeficiency are absent (however, many patients who are asymptomatic can have severe immunodeficiency and can benefit from antiretroviral and anti-*Pneumocystis* therapy)

Serologic Response (Enzyme Immunoassay)

Widely available and the primary diagnostic test

Defined sensitivity and specificity

Positive predictive value varies with prevalence of HIV infection in the population; usually requires confirmatory testing by Western blot, immunofluorescence, radioimmunoprecipitation, or recombinant viral proteins or synthetic peptides

A few persons may be infected with HIV-1 but may not seroconvert for prolonged periods

Antigen Detection

Solid-phase radioimmunoassay and antigen-capture enzyme immunoassay can detect 10 pg of p24 antigen per milliliter of serum

Amount of antigen varies with disease progression; in many populations only 10–50 percent of HIV-infected persons are positive; thus, sensitivity is low as a diagnostic tool in all but very selected populations

Viral Genome Detection by Hybridization

Investigational

0.01–0.001 percent of CD4+ T cells are positive for HIV RNA by hybridization

Sensitivity is improved by in vitro enzymatic amplification of the HIV proviral DNA by PCR; false-positive results may also occur

Virus Culture

Expensive, time-consuming, and available only in research laboratories

Highly specific (100 percent) and sensitive (>98 percent)

With current techniques it is the current "gold standard" for detecting latent infection

---

screening high-risk groups for HIV infection. Following the initial screening procedure, more-specific tests confirm the diagnosis.

To understand the basis for serologic testing, a brief review of the HIV antigens that produce the most consistent serologic response is helpful. HIV has three major structural genes—*gag, pol,* and *env*—each of which codes for one or more proteins expressed in infected cells or in the mature virus (see Chap. 4). The *gag* gene encodes the major core proteins, including p55, a polypeptide of 55 kDa, which is cleaved to form p24 and p18. The *pol* gene encodes three proteins: p66 and p51, both known to have reverse transcriptase activity, and the nuclease-integrase protein p31. The *env* gene encodes a glycoprotein of 160 kDa, gp160, which is cleaved into the surface glycoprotein gp120 and the transmembrane protein gp41. HIV-infected persons produce a spectrum of antibodies to all or some of these proteins.

The most commonly used assay to detect antibodies to HIV-1 is the enzyme-linked immunosorbent assay (ELISA), which detects antibodies to multiple viral proteins, because a whole-viral lysate is used as the target antigen. A prototype enzyme immunoassay procedure is shown in Fig. 5-1. Serum samples that the ELISA shows to be "initially reactive" are tested again to rule out technical errors. If the test is positive again, the sample is considered "repeatably reactive." To rule out false-positive results, these reactive specimens are then tested by a confirmatory method.

Clinical studies have shown that the ELISA has more than 99 percent sensitivity and specificity in both blood-donor and high-risk populations. The predictive value of a positive result, however, varies with the population tested, due to differences in the prevalence of the infection in low- and high-risk populations. For example, one commonly used immunoassay marketed by the Genetic Systems Corporation was evaluated using 9703 serum and plasma samples from blood donation centers from cities considered to have populations of both high and low risk for HIV infection. In the low-risk population, 21 specimens were repeatedly reactive and 14 of those were positive by a confirmatory method, demonstrating 100 percent sensitivity and 99.9 percent specificity. The predictive value of a positive enzyme immunoassay result in this population with low prevalence (less than 1 percent) of disease thus was 67 percent. In studies from 1414 patients from a high-risk group, the sensitivity of the assay compared with the confirmatory method was 99.9 percent (875 positive of 876 confirmatory positive) and the specificity was 99.9 percent (537 negative of 538 confirmatory negative). Because this population had a high prevalence of disease (66 percent), the assay's positive predictive value was 99.9 percent. In general, it is important to have a bimodal distribution of nonreactive and reactive results (i.e., no "gray area" of overlap between reactive and nonreactive results), independent of the population tested, to achieve maximum sensitivity and specificity in the ELISA. Several other commercial kits achieve similar sensitivity and specificity and are licensed for diagnostic testing by the U.S. Food and Drug Administration (FDA).

Compared with other test formats, the ELISA has the advantages of sensitivity, specificity, and ease of automation for reducing the time and

Figure 5-1.

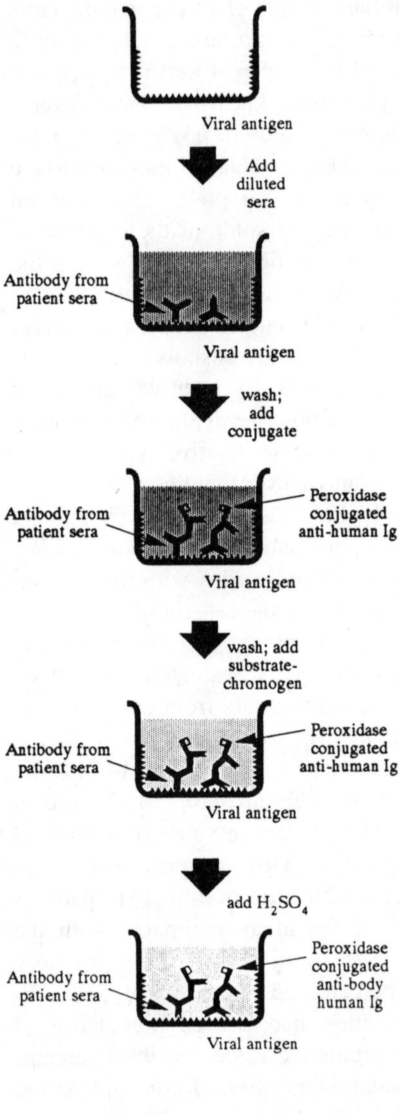

The purified, inactivated virus is adsorbed onto wells of a microwell plate.

Samples to be tested are diluted in sample diluent and added to each well, incubated with the adsorbed antigen and washed. If antibodies to the virus are present, they bind to antigen and are not removed by washing.

The conjugate reagent, peroxidase-labeled goat anti-human immunoglobulin, is then added to the wells and will bind to the antibody-antigen complex, if present. Unbound conjugate is removed by a wash step.

Next, chromogen reagent is added to the plate and allowed to incubate. A blue or blue-green color develops in proportion to the amount of antibody bound to the antigen-coated plate.

The addition of acid stops the enzyme reaction, resulting in a color change to yellow. The optical absorbance of controls and specimens is determined with a spectrophotometer with wavelength set at 450 nm.

cost. Several problems can occur, however, that may give false-positive or false-negative results. False-positive results can be due to reactions to cellular antigens in the cell line used to produce the virus, or due to circulating antibodies to human histocompatibility leukocyte antigen (HLA), nuclear antigens, and other cellular antigens in patients with autoimmune disease or lymphoproliferative disorders, in multiparous women, and in recipients of multiple transfusions (Table 5-2). False-negative results

Table 5-2. Frequency (percent) of false-positive ELISA reactivity in panels of serum specimens from patients with other immunologic abnormalities

Abnormality	Percent
Hematologic malignancy	0–7
DNA viral infections	5
Rheumatoid factor, antinuclear antibodies, other autoantibodies	17
Multiple myeloma	21
Primary biliary cirrhosis	20
Primary sclerosing cholangitis	12
Alcoholic hepatitis	13
Multiparous or multiply transfused persons with anti-HLA-DR4 antibodies	ND*

*ND = not determined.

Source: Adapted from Steckelberg JM, Cockeril III FR. Serologic testing for human immunodeficiency virus antibodies. *Mayo Clin Proc* 1988;63:373–380.

may be due either to decreased antibody associated with late-stage disease or to the lack of detectable antibody soon after initial infection.

Current enzyme immunoassay screens are designed to detect antibody to HIV-1. They do not reliably detect antibody to HIV-2 in blood from persons with HIV-2 infection because HIV-1 and HIV-2 exhibit antigenic cross-reactivity (mostly between *gag* and polymerase proteins and less between envelope proteins).

Confirmatory tests

After enzyme immunoassay screening, repeatedly reactive specimens are tested by a confirmatory method to ensure the specific reaction to the virus. Such methods include those that detect antibody to individual viral proteins, such as Western blot or radioimmunoprecipitation, and those that use infected cultured cells to detect antibody, such as immunofluorescence.

The Western blot (Fig. 5-2, graphic representation) is the most common method used to detect antibody response to specific HIV viral proteins. Purified HIV viral proteins are electrophoresed in sodium dodecyl sulfate (SDS) gels and transferred to nitrocellulose paper. The paper is then incubated with the serum sample, and specific antibody is detected with an enzyme-conjugated, antihuman antibody and enzyme substrate. Most human sera that contain antibodies to the virus react with a constellation of viral proteins representing envelope (gp160/120, gp41), core (p55, p24, p18), and polymerase (p66, p51, p31). A small percentage of sera reacts

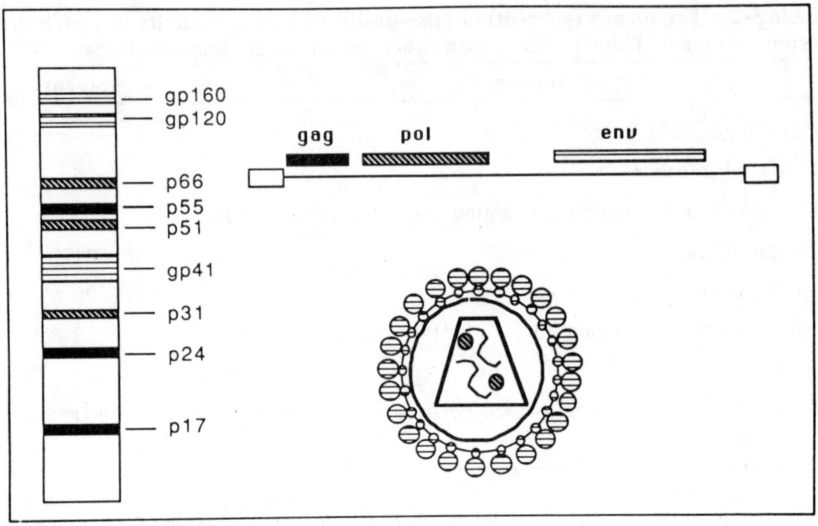

Figure 5-2. Graphic representation of an ideal HIV-1 immunoblot showing the relationship between the HIV genome, the translational protein products, the assembled virion, and the immunoblot pattern. The regulatory genes and their respective translational products are not shown.

only with single core proteins (e.g., p24). The specificity of antibodies to a single core protein of HIV and the significance of these reactions are uncertain; therefore, this reaction pattern is called *atypical* or *indeterminate*. In general, a Western blot is considered positive if a person demonstrates antibodies to any two of p24, gp41, and gp160/120 proteins.

The Western blot has demonstrated greater than 99 percent sensitivity and specificity, but the procedure is time-consuming and labor intensive. The use of the Western blot to confirm enzyme immunoassay results is especially important in populations with a low prevalence of infection.

Radioimmunoprecipitation is another method that detects antibody to specific viral proteins. HIV viral proteins are radiolabeled with amino acids, and lysates are incubated with the serum. Following washing procedures, the radiolabeled proteins that bind to the antibodies are electrophoresed on SDS gels and detected by autoradiography. This procedure is less adaptable to a clinical laboratory than the Western blot but may be more sensitive in detecting viral glycoproteins. It is mainly a research tool.

Indirect immunofluorescence is a third method of detecting HIV antibody. A serum sample is incubated with HIV-infected cells fixed to microscope slides. Specific antibody is detected by fluorescein-labeled, antihuman antibody, and positive cells are visualized using the fluorescence microscope. The method is as sensitive and specific as the Western blot in laboratories experienced in using this technique. It is relatively simple and inexpensive but, as with all immunofluorescent techniques, reading depends upon the person examining the slide, and the test can be subjective.

Second- and third-generation antibody assays

To develop more-sensitive and more-specific tests for HIV, second-generation assays have used recombinant DNA technology or synthetic peptide chemistry to detect antibodies to specific viral proteins. Viral glycoproteins encoded by the envelope gene (gp41) and core proteins from the *gag* gene (p24) have been expressed in *Escherichia coli* and have been used in enzyme immunoassay and Western blot assay formats. The recombinant proteins from the envelope region have shown greater than 99 percent sensitivity. However, because the antibody response to HIV is diverse, it is best to include viral proteins from both envelope and *gag* gene products. The immune response to the *gag* gene products is diverse, and most studies show lower sensitivity to the *gag* region recombinant proteins. An alternative approach is to use chemically synthesized peptides that represent immunodominant regions of the viral proteins. Synthetic peptides are not contaminated by bacterial proteins and may give more-specific reactions. A 25-amino-acid sequence from the gp41 protein of the virus has been shown to have greater than 99 percent sensitivity compared with the enzyme immunoassay and the Western blot.

Both recombinant proteins and synthetic peptides offer the advantages of low cost, safety, and manufacturing reliability. They also may be more sensitive and specific because the target antigens do not contain cellular contaminants present in many enzyme immunoassay tests that use whole-virus lysates. In addition, individual viral antigens can be used to detect antibody to separate viral proteins. This may be useful in determining the prognosis of seropositive persons, because individuals with AIDS-related complex (ARC) and AIDS appear to have a lower titer and a lower prevalence of antibodies to *gag* (p24). The absence of antibodies to *gag* has been shown to be associated with more rapid development of AIDS.

Several tests employing synthetic or recombinant-derived HIV antigens have been recently licensed by the FDA for confirmatory testing. As with the whole-virus lysate assays, these can be automated and run in an ELISA format. It is likely that many of these recombinant antigen assays will be utilized in the future as confirmatory tests instead of the Western blot, or as specific screening assays to replace whole-virus lysate assays.

Seroconversion

Antibody assays are useful for detecting past infection; however, there are instances in which a person may become infected and not possess measurable antibodies. This "window" period before antibody is detected occurs with all infections. For HIV, almost all patients develop detectable antibodies by the ELISA and Western blot assays by 6–12 weeks after infection (Fig. 5-3). Recently, however, in some patients, HIV-1 virus has been shown to be present in lymphocytes and macrophages by culture and DNA amplification procedures, but antibodies have not been detected. Some of these patients were followed for 12–18 months or longer before they seroconverted as detected by standard antibody assays. Several studies indicate that the percentage of patients who are HIV infected and exhibit this prolonged window is low (probably less than 3 percent of most populations); however, the frequency and host determinants of this prolonged latent infection are not well characterized. These findings do introduce an element of uncertainty in persons with negative antibody assays, especially if they are engaged in high-risk behaviors. To detect these patients requires the use of assays that will detect viral antigen, nucleic acid, or infectious virus.

DETECTION OF HIV ANTIGEN

Commercially available HIV-1 antigen assays may be useful for documenting HIV in infants or antibody-negative persons. However, these assays lack the sensitivity of virus culture. The most commonly utilized antigen assays

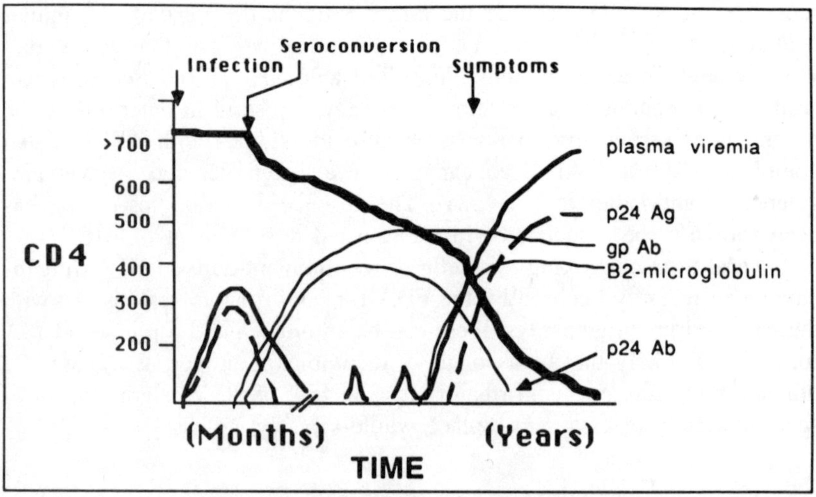

Figure 5-3. Relationship between CD4 T-cell count and clinical progression of HIV infection. Some of the other commonly used markers (both direct and indirect) of HIV replication are also shown.

detect HIV core antigens (p24) and use an antigen-capture immunoassay format in which specific anti-HIV antibody (monoclonal or polyclonal) is used to capture HIV antigen. Enzyme-labeled antibody to HIV and enzyme substrate are then used to detect the antibody-antigen complex.

The p24 antigen assays have been most widely utilized for detecting HIV-1 antigen in serum. Studies show that very early after infection, antigen is present for a short time in the serum before circulating antibodies develop to the envelope and then the core proteins. This period of antigenemia ranges from 2 weeks to 2 months or more; subsequently, antigen is cleared and antibodies to the core protein are detected. As disease progresses (years later), the level of HIV-p24 antigen increases and that of antibody to HIV-1 p24 antigen decreases (Fig. 5-3). About 50 percent of patients with AIDS possess HIV-p24 antigen in serum, compared to about 20 percent of patients who are asymptomatic but seropositive. Persons treated with the anti-HIV drug zidovudine (azidothymidine, AZT) may show a reduced amount of circulating antigen. The antigen test, therefore, is a useful way to measure potential in vivo antiviral chemotherapy.

DETECTION OF HIV NUCLEIC ACID

DNA probe technology for viral RNA and DNA is an alternative methodology for virus detection. By using various hybridization techniques, HIV sequences can be detected in the peripheral blood lymphocytes or tissues of about 50 percent of symptomatic, HIV-seropositive patients. (This contrasts to HIV culture, which has a sensitivity of greater than 97 percent.) By in situ hybridization, infected cells are observed at a very low frequency (less than 0.01 percent of the total mononuclear cells from the peripheral blood). This difference in sensitivity may be due to a small number of HIV genome copies per cell or to sampling error resulting from the extremely low frequency of cells expressing HIV. By employing in vitro enzymatic methods to amplify selective parts of the HIV genome [a process called *gene amplification,* using a technique termed *polymerase chain reaction (PCR)]*, the sensitivity of nucleic acid hybridization may approach that of virus culture. The gene amplification method also is amenable to automation and may decrease both the time and the cost of virus culture.

DETECTION OF HIV BY CULTURE

HIV is isolated in primary mixed lymphocyte culture (Fig. 5-4). Peripheral blood lymphocytes to be tested for the presence of HIV are separated from

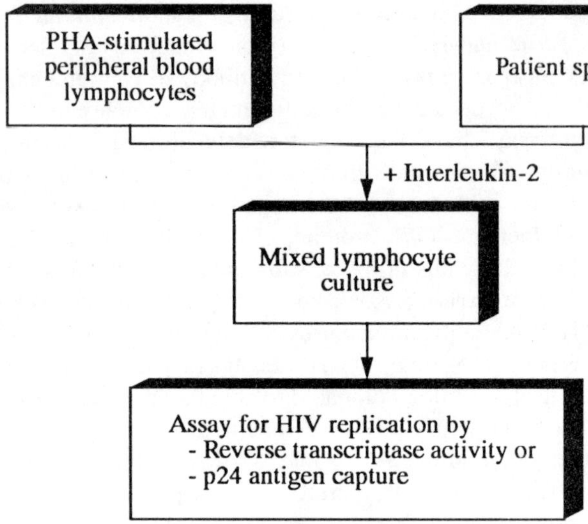

Figure 5-4. Procedure for HIV virus culture.

heparinized, fresh whole blood by ficoll-Hypaque density gradient centrifugation. The mononuclear cells are removed and cocultivated with phytohemagglutinin (PHA)-stimulated normal peripheral blood lymphocytes from HIV-seronegative donors. The PHA (a plant-derived mitogen) stimulates the normal CD4+ T cells to produce receptors for the lymphokine IL-2. In the presence of purified, exogenous IL-2, the CD4+ T cells further differentiate into blasts, which are more receptive to viral infection. Traces of PHA and the antigenic stimulation from the culture conditions are responsible for stimulating the expression of HIV in the patient's infected CD4+ mononuclear cells. Cultures are assayed for HIV production twice weekly and are incubated for at least 28 days before being considered negative. Other specimens, including serum, plasma, cerebrospinal fluid, genital secretions, and homogenized tissues, are cocultivated with normal donor lymphocytes by a similar procedure.

To detect HIV in culture, assays of the culture fluid for the HIV reverse transcriptase or HIV-1 p24 antigen are performed. An increase in either viral product over time reflects HIV replication. Because reverse transcriptase also is found in human retroviruses other than HIV (e.g., HTLV types I and II), cultures positive for reverse transcriptase activity require confirmation by electon microscopy, immunofluorescence, or p24 antigen capture. Production of a characteristic cytopathic effect (multinucleated giant cells) also may be used as a qualitative marker for HIV production. Most (80–90 percent) HIV-positive peripheral blood lymphocytes are usually detected by the second week of culture.

Isolation of HIV from different HIV-seropositive populations

HIV has been isolated not only from peripheral blood lymphocytes but also from tears, saliva, serum, plasma, breast milk, cerebrospinal fluid, brain, peripheral nerve, skin, semen, cervical secretions, and various internal organs. Although not all of these sources have been implicated in the epidemiologic transmission of infection, the CDC recommends that any seropositive person be considered infectious.

Current HIV culture technique isolates HIV from nearly all persons infected with HIV from their peripheral blood lymphocytes, and is the most sensitive and specific assay for documenting HIV infection. HIV can also be isolated from cell-free plasma of seropositive patients and from the plasma of asymptomatic patients (Fig. 5-5). Plasma virus titers increase with disease progression; therefore, plasma viremia is a marker of disease progression.

Because of cost and time constraints, HIV culture is a research supplement to the serologic diagnosis of HIV infection. There are, however, two potential applications for HIV culture in the clinical setting. First is the high-risk person with a suspected HIV infection (CDC group I) in whom a measurable antibody response has not occurred, either because the infection

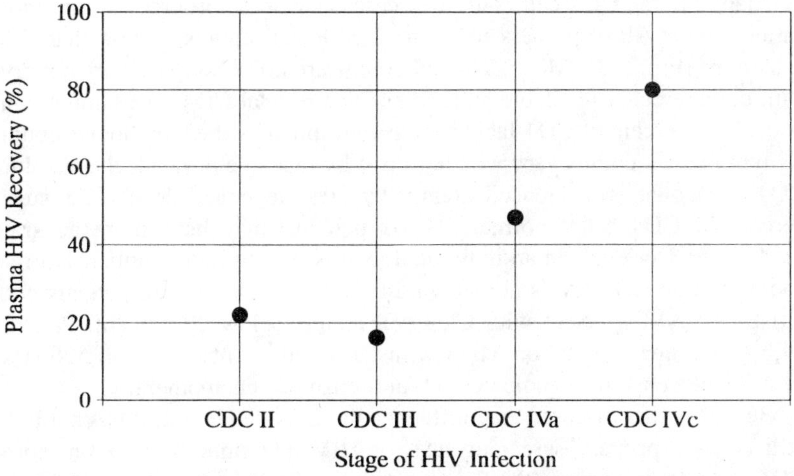

Figure 5-5. Recovery of plasma-associated HIV from patients with different stages of infection.
CDC group II: asymptomatic
CDC group III: persistent generalized lymphadenopathy
CDC group IVa: symptomatic (ARC)
CDC group IVc: opportunistic infections (AIDS)

is acute or because the person is unable to mount an immune response, as in the case of a patient with congenital hypogammaglobulinemia. (This also represents a potential application for viral antigen detection.) Second, the infant born to an HIV-seropositive mother will have maternal HIV IgG present for the first 6–15 months of life. Since accurate HIV IgM testing is not yet available, HIV culture, antigen detection, and HIV nucleic acid detection by PCR are useful tests for determining HIV infection in neonates (see Chap. 10). Culture and PCR are also useful for identifying the seronegative high-risk individual with latent infection.

INDIRECT MARKERS OF HIV DISEASE PROGRESSION

Indirect markers of HIV infection include the CD4 cell count, beta-2 microglobulin levels, and serum neopterin levels.

CD4 cell count

The CD4 cell count has been utilized most extensively in HIV-infected individuals and clinically is the most useful of these markers. As discussed in Chap. 11, the CD4 cell count decreases as disease progresses, and most patients with AIDS possess absolute CD4+ cell counts of less than 200 cells/mm^3 (Fig. 5-3). Most CD4 cell counts are done using flow cytometry, with commercially available antibodies. The normal CD4+ cell count consists of the percent of CD4-labeled cells multiplied by the lymphocyte count. As lymphocyte counts vary whether done by machine or hand, the absolute CD4 cell count is influenced greatly by these technical details. As such, percent of CD4 cells (normal, 31–61 percent) may be a more accurate marker of CD4 levels in an individual than is the absolute number. Normal and abnormal CD4 levels are shown in Table 5-3. Almost all patients with AIDS and ARC present with CD4 cell counts below 20 percent. Patients with symptomatic ARC or AIDS with CD4 cell counts less than 500 (less than 25 percent) are candidates for antiretroviral chemotherapy.

Because other diseases may influence the CD4 cell count, it has not been utilized as a primary screening test for HIV infection. In addition, some CD4 cells do not stain with all commercial anti-CD4 antibodies; hence, the CD4 cell count may be falsely low. A thorough analysis should include a complete profile of the T-lymphocyte subsets, that is, the percent T4 cells (CD4) and the percent T8 cells (CD8) should initially be determined. The normal percent of CD8 cells ranges from 18 to 39 percent; thus, the combined CD4 and CD8 subsets should be 80–90 percent of the total

Table 5-3. CD4 cell count (absolute numbers) and percent of total CD4 cell counts

No. cells/mm³	Percent
≥800 (normal)	40 (range, 31–61)
600	30
500	25
400	20
200	10
100	5
<100	<5

Note: Data obtained by using flow cytometric methods at the University of Washington, Seattle.

enumerated lymphocytes. B cells normally constitute 5–20 percent of the lymphocyte population.

In the HIV-positive patient, the CD4 cell count is useful in predicting disease progression, in deciding whether antiretroviral chemotherapy is indicated, and in determining whether an acute infection is likely to be due to an opportunistic pathogen (e.g., *Pneumocystis carinii*) or a community-acquired infection. For example, in HIV-infected patients with CD4 cell counts greater than 500/mm^3, *P. carinii* pneumonia (PCP) is unusual (Table 5-4). Therefore, an HIV-infected person with a high CD4 cell count is more likely to have pneumonia due to bacterial or mycobacterial (tuberculosis) infection than is a person with a low CD4 cell count.

Table 5-4. Percent of HIV-seropositive persons who develop PCP at 6, 12, and 36 months, by baseline CD4+ cell count

Baseline CD4+ cell count mm³	Percent of HIV-seropositive persons at 6 months	12 months	36 months
<200	8.4	18.4	33.3
201–350	0.5	4.0	22.9
351–500	0.0	1.4	9.0
501–700	0.0	0.4	8.3
>700	0.0	0.0	3.8

Source: Centers for Disease Control. Guidelines for prophylaxis against *Pneumocystis carinii* pneumonia for persons infected with human immunodeficiency virus. *MMWR* 1989;38(S-5):1–9.

Beta-2 microglobulin and neopterin

Beta-2 microglobulin is a plasma membrane protein associated with the light chain of the major histocompatibility class I molecule that is released by B cells, T cells, and monocyte-macrophages as a response to their activation. Studies have shown that patients with progressive HIV-1 infection have elevated levels (greater than 3 mg/ml) of beta-2 microglobulin. The sensitivity and specificity of this protein have not, however, been well evaluated in a wide cross section of patients. Sequential monitoring of beta-2 microglobulin has been shown to correlate with disease progression. As infection due to CMV also increases the beta-2 microglobulin level, it may be a less specific reflection of HIV activity than is the CD4 cell count.

Neopterin (6-D-*erythro*-trihydroxypropylpterin) is an intermediate product in the metabolism of guanosine-triphosphate; macrophages activated by antigen-stimulated T lymphocytes release neopterin. As such, neopterin levels are increased in the serum and urine of patients with AIDS and a number of other clinical conditions involving activation of cellular immunity.

CLINICAL UTILITY OF HIV TESTS

A variety of tests diagnostic for HIV can be used clinically. For example, a patient may report fatigue and weight loss to a physician. After taking a medical history, the physician determines that the patient is a member of a high-risk group for HIV infection. After consent is obtained, the patient's serum is tested by enzyme immunoassay for detection of antibody to HIV. If the serum is repeatably reactive by enzyme immunoassay, it is then tested by Western blot to confirm the presence of specific antibody to HIV viral proteins. If the result is positive, the patient is then counseled and followed for changes in clinical status. A CD4 cell count should be performed to stage the patient in the disease course and to see if he or she is a candidate for antiretroviral therapy. Tests for specific antibody to the core protein p24, or for the presence of the p24 core antigen, may also be useful in this staging process. If there is a lower titer of antibody to p24 or if antigen is present in serum, the patient may need closer monitoring for disease progression.

GUIDELINES FOR HIV ANTIBODY TESTING

Establishing the laboratory confirmation of HIV infection has two important functions: to establish a diagnosis and to interrupt transmission of the virus. Serologic testing combined with counseling can modify behavior and encourage low-risk sexual practices. To assist the clinician in deciding who would most benefit from serologic testing, we have outlined the current U.S. Public Health Service guidelines for HIV antibody testing (Table 5-5). In certain instances, we have made suggestions to increase the scope of testing; these suggestions should prompt the clinician to search for a history of a high-risk category and to obtain consent for HIV antibody testing. For early HIV infection (which could present as either an acute mononucleosis-like syndrome or acute aseptic meningitis), repeated serologic testing at 6, 9, and 24 weeks may be necessary because of the delayed antibody responses to HIV infection.

Table 5-5. Guidelines for HIV antibody testing

Decrease Transmission

All blood and organ (including semen) donors
Persons who consider themselves at risk for HIV infection
Persons with a sexually transmitted disease
IV drug users
Persons who received blood transfusions between 1978 and 1985
Women of childbearing age with identifiable risk for infection (including those planning surrogate motherhood)
Persons planning marriage where the seroprevalence is ⩾0.1 percent
Male and female prostitutes
Persons admitted to hospitals in those age groups deemed to have a high prevalence of HIV infection
Persons in correctional institutions (and perhaps institutions for chronic psychiatric care where regulation of sexual activity may be difficult and segregation may be necessary to protect seronegative persons)
Pregnant women

Diagnosis

Generalized lymphadenopathy
Unexplained dementia or encephalopathy
Chronic unexplained fever
Chronic unexplained diarrhea
Unexplained weight loss or wasting syndrome
Tuberculosis
Chronic candidiasis
Kaposi's sarcoma
Primary lymphoma of the brain
Generalized herpesvirus infection in a patient more than 1 month old
(Aseptic meningitis)*
(Unexplained interstitial pneumonia)
(Idiopathic thrombocytopenic purpura)
(Heterophile-negative infectious mononucleosis)*
(Unexplained psychosis or peripheral neuropathy)
(Any person with either a definitively or a presumptively diagnosed opportunistic infection, malignancy, or other disease consistent with AIDS)

(Continued)

Table 5-5. Guidelines for HIV antibody testing *(Continued)*

(Any infant born to a high-risk mother)†
For patients less than 13 years old
—Unexplained recurrent bacterial infections
—Lymphoid interstitial pneumonia or pulmonary lymphoid hyperplasia
—(Unexplained failure to thrive)
—(Unexplained developmental delay)
—(Unexplained parotitis)
—(Unexplained hepatitis)
—(Unexplained cardiomyopathy)

Note: Parenthetical guidelines are the authors' recommendations and depend on risk factors, age, and seroprevalence in the patient population.

*Caveat. For the initially HIV-seropositive person, serologic testing should be repeated at 6 weeks; if still negative, it should be repeated again at 3 and 6 months to exclude early infection.

†The presence of anti-HIV IgG by itself is insufficient evidence of HIV infection, because passively acquired maternal antibodies may persist for up to 15 months after birth. (Centers for Disease Control. Classification system for human immunodeficiency virus infection in children under 13 years of age. *MMWR* 1987;36:225–235.)

Source: Adapted from Centers for Disease Control. Public Health Service guidelines for counseling and antibody testing to prevent HIV infection and AIDS. *MMWR* 1987;36:509–515; and Centers for Disease Control. Revision of CDC case surveillance system for acquired immunodeficiency syndrome. *MMWR* 1987;36(15):3S–14S.

Although AIDS remains, for the most part, a clinical diagnosis, it is unusual under current clinical practice for a diagnosis to be confirmed without prior HIV serologic testing. However, in the absence of certain definitively diagnosed indicator diseases required by the current case definition, a positive serologic test for HIV antibody is required to confirm a diagnosis of AIDS in the following instances:

1. Definitively diagnosed disseminated coccidioidomycosis or histoplasmosis; isosporiasis; recurrent salmonella septicemia; extrapulmonary tuberculosis; disseminated mycobacterial disease caused by mycobacteria other than *Mycobacterium tuberculosis;* non-Hodgkin's lymphoma of high-grade pathologic type and of B-cell or unknown immunologic phenotype; Kaposi's sarcoma or primary lymphoma of the brain affecting patients who are less than 60 years old; dementia or encephalopathy; wasting syndrome; patients with syndromes indicative of AIDS, but who have received immunosuppressive or cytotoxic therapy within the 3 months prior to developing an indicator disease or who develop certain lymphoreticular malignancies within the 3-month period after developing an indicator disease; and patients with a genetic immunodeficiency syndrome or an acquired immunodeficiency syndrome atypical of HIV infection, such as hypogammaglobulinemia.

2. Presumptively diagnosed esophageal candidiasis, cytomegalovirus retinitis, PCP, Kaposi's sarcoma, toxoplasmosis of the brain affecting patients older than 1 month, and lymphoid interstitial pneumonia or pulmonary lymphoid hyperplasia in children less than 13 years old.

SUMMARY

Persons with HIV infection develop antibodies to several HIV-encoded proteins. The enzyme immunoassay currently used for screening blood donations and patient specimens detects antibody to multiple viral antigens and demonstrates greater than 99 percent sensitivity and specificity. In populations having a high prevalence of infection (e.g., 66 percent), the predictive value of a repeatably positive enzyme immunoassay is 99 percent. However, in populations with a low prevalence of infection (e.g., less than 1 percent), such as blood donors, the predictive value of a repeatably positive enzyme immunoassay is only about 60 percent. Other more specific methods, such as Western blot, immunofluorescence assay, or radioimmunoprecipitation, are used to confirm the presence of antibody to individual viral proteins in serum specimens that are repeatably positive by enzyme immunoassay.

Second-generation tests for antibody to specific viral proteins encoded by *env* and *gag* genes use either recombinant proteins produced in bacteria or chemically synthesized peptides. These tests are more specific than current enzyme immunoassays and are cheaper and safer to produce. Additionally, detection of antibodies to individual proteins may be important in monitoring disease progression.

Assays have been developed to detect viral antigens or viral RNA and DNA. Detection of viral antigen may be important early in infection, late in disease, and during antiviral chemotherapy. Virus culture and PCR also may be used to detect latent HIV infection.

There are several indirect markers of HIV infection that may be helpful for both disease staging and clinical management. For example, the CD4 cell count may be used for predicting disease progression and in deciding whether antiretroviral chemotherapy of *Pneumocystis carinii* prophylaxis are indicated.

Future development of laboratory tests for HIV detection must take into account the recent isolation and characterization of HIV-1 and other HIV types from Africa. Because HIV-1 and HIV-2 exhibit antigenic cross-reactivity mostly between *gag* and *pol* proteins and less between *env* proteins, HIV-2 may not be detected by current enzyme immunoassay screens that are based on detection of HIV-1 antibodies.

ADDITIONAL READING

Allain J-P, Paul DA, Senn D, Laurian Y. Serological markers in early stages of human immunodeficiency virus infection in haemophiliacs. *Lancet* 1986;8518:1233–1236.

Barre-Sinoussi F, Chermann J-C, Rey F, Nugeryre MT, et al. Isolation of a T lymphotropic retrovirus from a patient at risk for acquired immune deficiency syndrome (AIDS). *Science* 1983;220:868–871.

Centers for Disease Control. Classification system for human immunodeficiency virus (HIV) infection in children under 13 years of age. *MMWR* 1987;36:225–235.

Centers for Disease Control. Guidelines for prophylaxis against *Pneumocystis carinii* pneumonia for persons infected with human immunodeficiency virus. *MMWR* 1989;38(S-5):1–9.

Centers for Disease Control. Public Health Service guidelines for counseling and antibody testing to prevent HIV infection and AIDS. *MMWR* 1987;36:509–515.

Centers for Disease Control. Revision of CDC case surveillance system for acquired immunodeficiency syndrome. *MMWR* 1987;36(1S):3S–14S.

Chang NT, Huang J, Ghrayeb J, McKinney S, Chanda PK, Chang TW, Putney S, Sarngadharan MG, Wong-Staal F, Gallo RC. An HTLV-III peptide produced by recombinant DNA is immunoreactive with sera from patients with AIDS. *Nature* 1985;315:151–154.

Coombs RW, Collier AC, Allain JP, Nikora B, Leuther M, Gjerset GF, Corey LC. Plasma viremia in human immunodeficiency virus infection. *N Engl J Med* 1989;321:1626–1631.

Gallo RC, Sarin PS, Geimann EP, Robert-Guroff M, Richardson E, et al. Isolation of human T cell leukemia virus in acquired immune deficiency syndrome (AIDS). *Science* 1983;220:865–867.

Gallo D, Diggs JL, Shell GR, Dailey PJ, Hoffman MN, Riggs JL. Comparison of detection of antibody to the acquired immune deficiency syndrome virus by enzyme immunoassay, immunofluorescence, and Western blot methods. *J. Clin Micro* 1986;23:1049–1051.

Imagawa DT, Lee M, Wolinsky SM, et al. Human immunodeficiency virus type 1 infection in homosexual men who remain seronegative for prolonged periods. *N Engl J Med* 1989;320:1458–1462.

McDougal JS, Cort SP, Kennedy MS, Cabridilla CD, Feorino PM, Francis DP, Hicks D, Kalyanaraman VS, Martin LS. Immunoassay for the detection and quantitation of infectious human retrovirus lymphadenopathy-associated virus (LAV). *J Immunol Meth* 1985;76:171–183.

Sarngadharan MG, Popovic M, Bruch L, Schupbach J, Gallo RC. Antibodies reactive with human T lymphotropic retroviruses (HTLV-III) in the serum of patients with AIDS. *Science* 1984;224:506–508.

Steckelberg JM, Cockeril FR III. Serologic testing for human immunodeficiency virus antibodies. *Mayo Clin Proc* 1988;63:373–380.

Stramer SL, Heller JS, Coombs RW, Parry JV, Ho DD, Allain JP. Markers of HIV infection prior to IgG antibody seropositivity. *JAMA* 1989;262:64–69.

6

HIV: Screening and Counseling Guidelines

Connie Celum
Robert W. Wood

Testing for HIV is an issue of considerable medical and social complexity. Although the laboratory procedures are relatively inexpensive, accurate, and highly predictive among persons at risk for HIV, AIDS and HIV infection are associated with almost unprecedented stigma. HIV infection, furthermore, is lifelong, incurable, and, despite antidiscrimination laws and civil rights judgments, carries the potential for discrimination, in housing, employment, and restrictions in insurance, immigration, and travel. Careless release of even the fact that a person sought HIV testing can cause irreparable harm. Many at risk for this infection are understandably reluctant to learn whether they have acquired the virus, and some will decline testing.

We present a primary care practitioner's approach to HIV testing and specifically include (1) how and whom to screen for the risk of HIV, (2) how to evaluate the risk of HIV infection, (3) when to recommend testing, (4) the pros and cons of testing, (5) the interpretation of HIV tests, and (6) how to provide pre- and posttest counseling.

WHEN TO CONSIDER HIV TESTING

When the patient requests the test or presents with HIV-related findings

In view of intense media attention to AIDS, it is not surprising that many patients request HIV testing as a chief complaint. In fact, a patient's anxiety about the risk of AIDS may take the form of a present illness. Physicians can serve their patients best by first convincing themselves that a reasonable risk of HIV infection exists before carrying out HIV testing, which is not without potential adverse consequences. A reasonable threshold of infection likelihood should be reached before testing is recommended, as with decisions to perform other expensive or potentially risky tests. Clinicians do not have to comply when, for example, patients request penicillin for a sore throat or diazepam for problems of daily life. Clinical criteria for HIV testing should be applied to ensure quality care and because of potential legal consequences. Nonetheless, for many low-risk patients who request testing, the anxiety-reducing benefit of a negative test result often outweighs the small risk of a false-positive or indeterminate result.

Medical indications for HIV testing

HIV testing should be recommended for persons with symptoms or signs suggestive of HIV infection if there is reason to believe that they may be infected (e.g., they have engaged in high-risk behavior or have been exposed to potentially infected blood or blood products). Suggestive manifestations include an illness of more than 2 weeks' duration that is unexplained by common evaluation; specific symptoms may include persistent fever, night sweats, persistent cough, dyspnea, diarrhea, fatigue, weight loss, lumps (skin or nodal), or neurologic symptoms (headaches, sensory or motor symptoms, cognitive changes). Signs suggestive of HIV infection include tachypnea, skin lesions (Kaposi's sarcoma), persistent viral rash, persistent or widespread herpes zoster in a young person, fundoscopic abnormalities, mouth disease (thrush, severe gingivitis, hairy leukoplakia, Kaposi's sarcoma), generalized lymphadenopathy or splenomegaly, and otherwise unexplained neurologic signs. Beyond signs and symptoms of disease, opportunistic diseases suggestive of altered cellular immunity or diagnoses such as tuberculosis or interstitial pneumonia should alert practitioners to the possibility of HIV infection (see Chap. 8).

Because of accumulating evidence of the value of drugs (e.g., zidovudine, inhaled pentamidine) in preventing or delaying morbidity in HIV-infected persons (see Chap. 11), HIV testing of persons at risk can be medically important. Seropositive persons, furthermore, need immunologic evaluation to define levels of immune function and eligibility for drug therapy.

HIV testing of individuals at increased risk

In addition to medical indications for HIV testing, public health officials recommend that persons at risk for HIV infection undergo counseling and voluntary testing. The CDC recommends that persons seeking evaluation and treatment for STDs, prostitutes, and persons in correctional institutions be counseled to undergo voluntary testing because they are at increased risk for HIV infection. Testing should be considered for men who have had sex with prostitutes, for individuals with many sexual partners, for persons from countries where heterosexual transmission is common, and for others at risk. The CDC also recommends, and several states require, that all women seeking prenatal care undergo screening or testing for HIV infection. Screening includes obtaining a history of risk factors for HIV infection and assessing an individual for symptoms or signs of infection. If a risk of infection is identified, voluntary HIV antibody testing should be recommended. Common laboratory tests such as complete blood cell counts may reveal neutropenia, lymphopenia, or other abnormalities suggestive of HIV infection.[1] These findings have variable predictive value depending on the probability of HIV infection determined when the history is obtained.

Most public health officials do not recommend HIV testing for everyone or for all persons seeking a marriage license or entering a hospital. Despite the highly sensitive and specific tests available to identify HIV carriers, testing of low- and no-risk populations is not cost effective and could result in a substantial number of persons being labeled falsely as HIV infected. Nevertheless, the federal government has implemented mandatory, broad-based testing for certain groups, including those in the military, those seeking to enter the military or the Job Corps, and those in the federal corrections system. Some states have mandated testing for state prisoners, sexual offenders, or IV drug users.

Requests for a second opinion

Increasingly, patients who request testing seek a second opinion, having been previously tested for risk, health, or screening purposes. In such situations, health care providers should evaluate the reasons for past tests the nature of the tests previously performed, and their results. Interpretation of previous test results must be based both on an assessment of the risk of infection (e.g., based on the risk history) and on specific test(s) previously performed. Risks for HIV acquisition since the earlier test and potential current contraindications also need to be considered before testing is repeated because risk behaviors are dynamic and may change over time.

Screening for HIV in patients who present for other reasons

Not all persons who might be counseled appropriately to consider HIV testing specifically request it. Many (perhaps most) present with other health-related complaints or for routine preventive care and are reluctant to discuss their sexual and drug-use behaviors. Therefore, all clinicians require skills to elicit a history of such behaviors.[2] Ideally, all practitioners, especially those who provide primary care, should know their patients' medical histories (including conditions such as STDs), sexual behaviors, and drug usage.

Relative contraindications for HIV testing

Except when testing is required independent of risk, testing should generally not be performed on persons who have no plausible source of exposure (e.g., anxious persons with no history of sexual, drug, or blood-product risk since the mid-1970s). Tests for HIV infection are not as reliable in low- or no-risk populations, and although false-positive and indeterminate test results are uncommon, they may constitute a substantial proportion of positive results in low-risk populations.

Candidates for testing may be depressed because of their HIV risk or coexistent disease. They may not be able to deal with the stress of actual testing or with a potentially positive or indeterminate test result. Unless diagnostic testing is urgent for medical management, these individuals should be advised to wait until they can cope better with the process and the result. Experience from the Seattle-King County AIDS Prevention Project suggests that 1–2 percent of high-risk clients who seek testing fall into this category and need to be referred for appropriate counseling prior to testing. Suicides after HIV testing have been reported anecdotally.

Dementia and delirium are relative contraindications to testing. Dementia is most common in persons with HIV infection in the final stages of AIDS, when testing is less useful, but it may appear earlier. Symptoms of the AIDS dementia complex, however, may be partially reversed with high-dose zidovudine therapy; HIV testing may therefore be useful for diagnostic and therapeutic purposes in an at-risk person with dementia. Delirium (by definition at least partially reversible) may be associated both with HIV infection and with risk behaviors, such as IV and recreational drug use, including crack cocaine, and alcohol abuse. In addition, some persons with significant mental illnesses, such as schizophrenia and depression, fixate on HIV infection or AIDS as solutions to or explanations for their problems and request that they be tested or treated for HIV and AIDS. When testing is necessary in mentally incompetent persons, consent should be obtained from a legal guardian after pretest counseling.

HIV TESTS

HIV antibody testing usually is done using the ELISA. If reactive, the ELISA is repeated on the same specimen. If this assay also is positive, confirmatory testing is performed. The HIV ELISA is a highly sensitive (at least 99 percent) and specific (99 percent) assay that detects antibodies to HIV viral proteins[3] (see Chap. 5). When used for public health or screening indications, an ELISA should be repeated on the same specimen to eliminate laboratory error. The positive predictive value of the ELISA—the likelihood that a positive test represents true HIV infection—is dependent on the prior probability of HIV infection in an individual (based on HIV risk factors and the prevalence of HIV in that risk group) and on the optical density of the ELISA result. It is important to perform a confirmatory test to ensure the accuracy of the results. These issues are discussed at length in Chap. 5. Figure 6-1 presents a simplified overview of HIV testing and interpretation.

A repeatedly reactive ELISA result should be followed by a more specific confirmatory test. The most commonly used confirmatory test is the Western blot, although some laboratories use immunofluorescent antibody or other tests (Chap. 5). The Western blot detects specific antibodies to viral antigens and is considered positive if antibody is detected to p24 and to gp41 or gp160/120, indeterminate if bands are present that do not meet the positive criteria, or negative if bands are absent. The Western blot is also reported to have 99 percent sensitivity and specificity when performed under optimal laboratory conditions. Nevertheless, indeterminate Western blot results are reported in low- and high-risk persons in as many as 25 percent of ELISA-reactive specimens, depending on the population screened and the specific Western blot assay used.[4] In low-risk individuals, indeterminate results are thought to result most commonly from the presence of autoantibodies or from cross-reactivity with antibodies to other viruses. In high-risk individuals, an indeterminate result often reflects a partial antibody response to HIV during seroconversion and can often be resolved as positive by repeating the Western blot in 3–6 months.

False-negative tests can occur in high-risk individuals, most often when the tests are performed early after infection with HIV (i.e., less than 6 months after exposure). Although some reports have documented latency periods of up to 3 years before the Western blot test became positive, almost all persons with HIV infection develop antibodies within 6 months.[5] One series with a 3-year follow-up found positive HIV cultures of blood mononuclear cells in 31 (23 percent) of 131 seronegative homosexual men who continued unprotected receptive rectal intercourse with multiple partners. Only 4 of the 31 infected men eventually seroconverted 11–18 months after

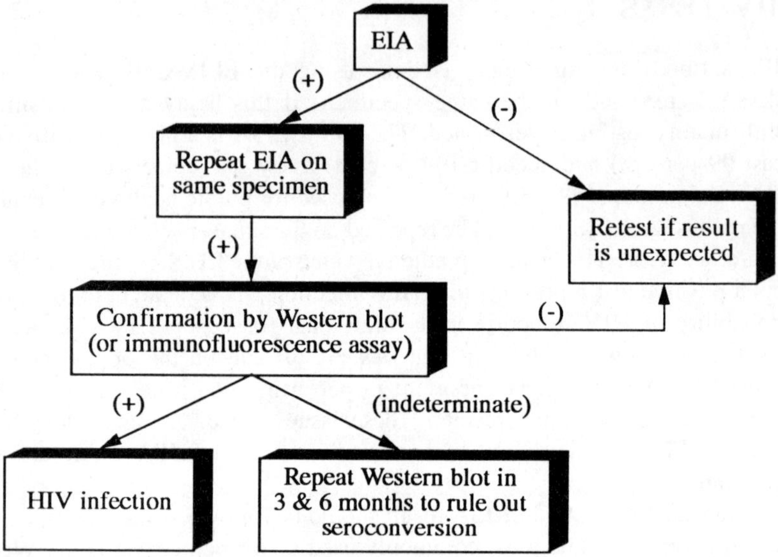

Figure 6-1. Simplified approach to the performance and interpretation of HIV antibody tests.

HIV was isolated.[6] This finding has not been reported in other cohorts of seronegative homosexual men and needs verification. Most people with negative results by ELISA but with documented exposure to HIV should be retested over a 6- to 12-month period and counseled intensively regarding safe sex and drug-use behaviors.

False-positive results represent a small proportion of reactive HIV serologic tests in persons at risk, but a higher proportion of positive tests in persons at no risk or very low risk for HIV infection. A repeatedly reactive result by ELISA followed by a positive Western blot signifies true HIV infection up to 99 percent of the time in high-risk individuals and 93–99 percent of the time in low-risk individuals.[7, 8] It has been estimated that fewer than 1 in 100,000 persons tested by both ELISA and Western blot will be falsely labeled as infected with HIV. Nevertheless, in the army's testing of 135,187 low-risk applicants for military service, 1 of 15 combined positive ELISA and Western blot specimens was considered false positive when supplemental tests, such as recombinant assays and radio-immunoprecipitation assays, were used to confirm positive ELISA and Western blot results.[8] In view of the military's excellent quality control and detailed multistep algorithm for identifying HIV-seropositive individuals, the false-positive rate might be lower than in some other settings. Most false-positive results probably are due to laboratory error. Given the low (20 percent) positive predictive value of a positive ELISA result in low- to no-risk populations, such patients should not be told their test results until both the ELISA and the confirmatory test results are available.

PRETEST COUNSELING AND INFORMED CONSENT

Informed consent is almost universally recommended when HIV testing is done; in many states it is illegal to perform HIV testing without informed consent, except when testing is legally mandated. In some states, informed consent need not be in writing, but discussion and verbal consent always should be documented in the medical record. Despite these recommendations, there is evidence from Minnesota[9] and numerous anecdotal reports which suggest that HIV testing commonly occurs without adequate counseling or true informed consent.

When a nonanonymously tested patient is documented as HIV infected, the physician normally is obligated to inform the patient. (This is a regulation for programs using federal funding to support testing and counseling.) In effect, a patient may not change his or her mind about learning his or her HIV infection status after the test is performed. This should be made clear during pretest counseling.

Counseling and communication skills are important in the setting of HIV testing to gain the client's trust and confidence; to convey information about the disease, its transmission, and test efficacy; to understand the reasons the patient is seeking HIV testing; and to evaluate the likelihood of infection. Although many individuals who present for HIV screening are quite knowledgeable about AIDS and HIV, this should not be assumed. The health care provider should cover numerous issues in pretest counseling (Table 6-1).

Risk assessment

After providing general education about HIV, AIDS, and the antibody test, one should determine why the individual seeks HIV testing. It is also important to ask about specific sexual and drug behaviors. Questions designed to explore such behaviors and past experiences should be sensitive, open-ended, and nonjudgmental, and should use vernacular language that the patient understands (see Chap. 12). It is essential to remember that some men consider themselves heterosexual despite a history of homosexual relationships, and some individuals who have homosexual attractions and consider themselves gay have never engaged in high-risk behavior.[10]

Similarly, questions to drug users need to be nonjudgmental and to employ the appropriate vernacular. A history of drug use should include

Table 6-1. Components of HIV pretest counseling

Component	Content

Education	Modes of HIV transmission
	  Intimate (see Chap. 1)
	
	Methods of reducing risk
	  Abstinence or mutual monogamy with an uninfected partner
	  Reduced number of sexual partners
	  Avoidance of anal receptive intercourse
	  Use of latex condoms with all forms of intercourse (preferably with a nonoxynol-9-spermicide)
	  Avoidance of IV drugs (especially sharing needles and syringes)
	  Use of a full-strength bleach solution if reusing or sharing needles or syringes
	
	HIV tests
	  Nature, purpose, consequences
	  Results: positive, indeterminate, negative
	  Options: anonymous, confidential
	  "Window" of seronegativity
	  Retesting
	
	HIV infection and AIDS
	  Difference between infection and AIDS
	  Partner notification
	  Risk of developing AIDS
	  Value of monitoring immune status
	  Treatment
	
	Physician's reporting requirements, if applicable

Evaluation	Risk (see Table 6-2) Coping ability Support systems

injected drugs, as well as alcohol, marijuana, and cocaine (including smoking free-base cocaine or crack) because of the influence on sexual behavior and the likelihood of engaging in unsafe sex while intoxicated or in trade for drugs. If an individual does inject drugs, knowing the frequency of use, specific drugs, previous places of use, and whether or not needles or syringes were shared is important. For example, needle sharing in New York or Miami is riskier than it is in Denver or San Francisco because of differences in the prevalence of HIV infection in IV drug users. Users of IV cocaine sometimes inject themselves as frequently as every 30 minutes to sustain a high; they dramatically increase their likelihood of HIV infection due to multiple potential exposures if they share needles or syringes.

Although some candidates for testing deny the highest risk behaviors (male-male sexual contact, IV drug use), increasing numbers have sexual exposure to someone from a high-risk group. This can be determined by asking, "Have you had sex with men who have sex with men, IV drug users, or people who have received blood?" Table 6-2 outlines the important information to obtain in assessing a person's risk for HIV infection.

Risks and benefits of HIV testing and assessment of coping skills

The decision to be tested for HIV infection is based on weighing the benefits and risks of testing. The benefits include relief of anxiety if the test result is negative, reinforcement of safe sex practices, important information for a high-risk woman contemplating pregnancy, assistance in diagnosing a high-risk person with possible symptoms or manifestations of HIV infection, and early monitoring of immune function and treatment for seropositive individuals. The risks include increased anxiety, relationship difficulties, possible discrimination, and the potential that seronegative individuals will use a negative result to justify continued or increased risky behavior.

The risk-benefit ratio has shifted with the recent results of the AIDS Clinical Trials Group studies in which zidovudine was found to substantially delay the progression of disease in asymptomatic, HIV-seropositive individuals with CD4 (helper) lymphocytes less than 500/mm^3 and individuals with moderate ARC. HIV testing and monitoring of CD4 lymphocytes are important in determining when to recommend zidovudine treatment. The patient must decide whether to be tested for HIV antibodies, but the provider can play an important role in discussing the pros and cons of testing with the patient, given the particular situation.

It is important to discuss the patient's actions if the test result is positive, that is, with whom he or she would discuss the results, and how the individual would respond in terms of sexual behavior, drug use, and suicide potential. If a patient appears psychotic or suicidal or does not have an adequate social support system, it is preferable to refer him or her for psychological counseling and defer HIV testing until the patient can cope better with the test result, especially if the patient has a high risk of being seropositive.

Confidentiality, reporting, and partner notification

As described in Chap. 3, some states require reporting of the identities of persons found to be HIV seropositive. Otherwise, it is important to maintain strict confidentiality of test results. Pretest counseling also must include informing the patient about the physician's intent or obligations concerning

Table 6-2. Components of pretest counseling for risk assessment for HIV infection

Component	Content
Sexual contacts	Number of partners Type: bisexual or homosexual men prostitutes, male or female IV drug users
Sexual practices	Type of intercourse: oral, anal-genital, genital-genital, with or without ejaculation Frequency Condom use, history of breakage
Drug use	Injected drugs (heroin, cocaine, ritalin) Frequency and duration Geographic locales (e.g., New York City) Sharing of needles or syringes HIV status of the needle-sharing partner
Known HIV exposure	Sexually or via an infected, needle-sharing partner
Hospitalizations, blood transfusions	Between 1977 and 1985

reporting to health authorities and partner notification. Anonymous testing and counseling services are offered in many settings, and whether to be tested confidentially or anonymously is a common concern of individuals seeking HIV testing. Confidential testing means including the HIV test results in the patient's chart with information that identifies that patient. The test result is then available to other health care professionals who are involved in the patient's care and have access to the record. Some physicians have elected to provide anonymous and confidential services.

POSTTEST COUNSELING

The follow-up interview to discuss test results should be scheduled at the time of pretest counseling and testing to reduce second guessing of antibody status by the patient. For persons at risk, and ideally in all situations, posttest counseling should occur in person, not by mail or telephone. Table 6-3 outlines the components of posttest counseling.

The test result should be communicated clearly and early in the posttest interview, in view of the anxiety that most patients experience. After the patient is informed of the test result, he or she should be given an opportunity to express feelings and ask questions. Communication of a positive result can be very difficult for both the provider and the patient; it is best if

Table 6-3. Components of HIV posttest counseling

Component	Content
Communication	Serologic test results
Interpretation of results	Positive: person is infected and infectious; does not mean that the person has AIDS Negative: no antibodies to HIV detected Indeterminate: antibody reactivity present; could be due to cross-reacting antibodies or early seroconversion
Follow-up plan (in general)	Repeat test: If the positive result is questioned or if the patient continues to deny high-risk behavior In 3–6 months for high-risk individuals with possible HIV exposure in the past 6 months In 3 and 6 months if the Western blot is indeterminate Reinforce the need for ongoing safe sex and drug-use practices Assess patients' understanding of the significance of the test result
(For newly diagnosed, HIV-seropositive individual)	Medical care (see Chap. 7) Psychological care [assess anxiety, depression, suicide risk, refer for counseling if indicated (see Chap. 12)] Partner notification, if appropriate Education to prevent transmission of HIV (e.g., no blood, organ, or semen donation; no sharing of toothbrushes or razors; safe sex and drug-use practices) Counseling regarding likelihood of progression to symptomatic HIV infection Referral for drug treatment (for IV drug or crack cocaine users)

the same physician who provided pretest counseling discusses the positive test result with the patient.

After the patient has had an opportunity to express his or her feelings, it is important to reiterate that a positive test result means that the individual has been infected with HIV and is infectious, but it does not mean that the patient has AIDS. The chance of becoming significantly symptomatic (about 50 to 70 percent over 10 years) and the effects of zidovudine and prophylaxis for opportunistic infections on improving survival and the quality of life need to be emphasized to underscore that seropositive individuals can have hope.

Before concluding the session, the provider should assess the patient's understanding of the positive result by asking what it means to the patient and what he or she plans to do with the result. In particular, the provider should reassess the suicide risk and discuss partner notification. Given the difficulty of assimilating information after receiving distressing news, it is helpful to schedule a follow-up interview to review this information and to reassess the patient's psychological status. Ideally, these sessions should be combined with further clinical evaluation (see Chap. 7), which usually will require several office visits.

Often it may be best to defer particularly difficult issues such as partner notification to the second interview (detailed in Chap. 3). The patient should be encouraged to discuss the test result with the physician or to establish a primary care relationship elsewhere if the physician is not the primary care provider. Patients should be referred for psychological counseling if there is severe anxiety or depression about the positive result or an inadequate social support system. Seropositive persons (and zero negative persons at substantial risk) should be told that they must not donate blood, semen, or body organs and that personal hygiene items (e.g., razors and toothbrushes) should not be shared. The importance of safe sex practices to avoid transmitting the virus to others should be reinforced, and the patient should be reminded of the obligation to inform future prospective partners of his or her infection.

A negative test should be interpreted based on the patient's level of risk. If the patient is at low risk, reassurance can be offered. The need for ongoing safer sex practices (and safe drug-use habits, if applicable) nevertheless should be strongly reinforced. If an individual has a history of possible recent or ongoing exposure to HIV, he or she should be encouraged to have testing repeated after 3–6 months. For individuals with an indeterminate Western blot result, the provider can explain that causes other than HIV are associated with indeterminate results and can recommend follow-up testing by ELISA and Western blot in 3–6 months.

SUMMARY

HIV testing presents challenges to health care providers that include: probing sensitive areas of personal behavior; communicating information about which people have anxiety and fears; assisting individuals in deciding whether HIV testing is recommended; interpreting positive, negative, and indeterminate results in the context of risk status; and counseling individuals about serologic status and risk reduction. The patient-provider interaction provides a unique and important opportunity to educate and counsel individuals about HIV infection and AIDS and about methods for reducing the likelihood of future infection with HIV.

REFERENCES

1. Wood R, Seattle-King County Department of Public Health, AIDS Prevention Project, unpublished data, 1989.
2. Brown H. *Familiar faces; hidden lives: The story of homosexual men in America today*. New York: Harcourt, Brace, Jovanovich, 1976.
3. Centers for Disease Control. Update. Serologic testing for antibodies to human immunodeficiency virus. *MMWR* 1988;36:833–840.
4. HIV Biotech/Dupont Western blot package insert, May 1987.
5. Ranki A, Krohn M, Allain J-P, et al. Long latency precedes overt seroconversion in sexually-transmitted HIV infection. *Lancet* 1987;ii:590–593.
6. Imagawa DT, Lee MT, Wolinsky SM, et al. Human immunodeficiency virus type 1 (HIV-1) infection in homosexual men who remain seronegative for prolonged periods. *N Engl J Med* 1989;320:1458–1462.
7. McDonald KL, Jackson JB, Bowman RJ, et al. Performance characteristics of serological tests for human immunodeficiency virus type 1 (HIV-1) antibody among Minnesota blood donors. *Ann Intern Med* 1989;110:617–621.
8. Burke DS, Brundage JF, Redfield RR, et al. Measurement of the false-positive rate in a screening program for human immunodeficiency virus infections. *N Engl J Med* 1988;319:961–964.
9. Henry K, Maki M, Crowley K. Analysis of the use of HIV antibody testing in a Minnesota Hospital. *JAMA* 1988;259:229–332.
10. Owens W. The clinical approach to the homosexual patient. *Ann Intern Med* 1980(I);93:90–92.

7

Management of HIV Infection in the Seropositive, Asymptomatic Patient

Frederick M. Hecht
John Jewett
William B. Bateman, Jr.

The discovery of HIV as the cause of AIDS, followed by the subsequent development of an antibody test to detect HIV infection, has defined a new category in the spectrum of AIDS-related illness: HIV-seropositive but asymptomatic.

There is suggestive evidence that in some patients the natural course of HIV infection can be favorably altered at this stage by treatment with zidovudine. It is clear that patients want to maximize their chances of remaining healthy and that current knowledge strongly suggests that several interventions are likely to be of benefit. Also relevant to the care of patients in this stage of HIV infection is the fact that knowledge of seropositivity is a difficult emotional burden. In addition, it is important to note that this group, estimated to number from 1 to 1.5 million, is the major reservoir for new HIV infection.

For these reasons, care of the HIV-seropositive, asymptomatic individual should aim to prevent morbidity and mortality, provide emotional support for the patient, and attempt to decrease spread of the virus. In addressing these goals, the following aspects of care require attention:

1. Initial biomedical evaluation to determine whether a patient is truly asymptomatic and to gather baseline information.

2. Ongoing screening for disease progression and opportunistic infections.
3. Initiation of prophylaxis.
4. Identification and strengthening of psychological and social supports.
5. Prevention of HIV transmission.
6. Encouragement of a healthy lifestyle.

Specific methods for addressing these issues are changing rapidly as research and clinical experience with different populations provide new information. We describe an approach to the care of the HIV-seropositive, asymptomatic patient that is based on a review of the medical literature and clinical experience.

INITIAL BIOMEDICAL EVALUATION AND SCREENING FOR DISEASE PROGRESSION

The initial evaluation of the apparently asymptomatic, HIV-seropositive patient must demonstrate whether the patient is truly free of signs and symptoms of disease. Follow-up of this evaluation is a means of identifying disease progression and of detecting opportunistic infections early. While the importance of baseline data in all areas of medical care is poorly documented and controversial, all physicians have had the experience of using the results of a previous test to interpret a current test result. Data gathered in this initial assessment are potentially useful in this manner.

History and physical examination

In taking an initial history from patients with HIV infection, one must be certain to include the sexual history, drug history, social networks and supports, and a history of exposure to tuberculosis or a positive tuberculin skin test. A review of systems, tailored to HIV infection, is presented in Table 7-1.

The physical examination of patients with HIV infection should include special attention to the areas listed in Table 7-2. Certain portions of the examination may need to be repeated only in response to specific complaints, but others should be repeated at least every 6 months to detect early signs of opportunistic infections or HIV-related malignancies. The latter category includes fundoscopy; lymph node, oral, and skin examinations; and body weight.

Table 7-1. Review of systems, symptoms, and possible causes in HIV-positive asymptomatic adults

System	Symptom	Possible causes
General	Fatigue, weight loss	AIDS-related wasting syndrome
	Fever, night sweats	TB, MAI, lymphoma, secondary syphilis
Dermatologic	Skin discoloration, rash, or eruption	Seborrheic dermatitis, Kaposi's sarcoma, herpes zoster or simplex, molluscum contagiosum, psoriasis
Oral	White areas	Oral candidiasis, hairy leukoplakia
	Ulcers	HSV, CMV
	Odynophagia	CMV, esophageal candidiasis, HSV
Visual	Visual deficits	CMV or toxoplasma retinitis
Cardiopulmonary	Persistent cough, dyspnea	PCP, TB, CMV pneumonia
Hematologic	Easy bruising	ITP
Gastrointestinal	Diarrhea	Bacterial or parasitic infection
	Anal pain	HSV, Kaposi's sarcoma, CMV
Genitourinary	Genital sores	Primary syphilis, chancroid, HSV
	Dysuria or penile discharge	Gonorrhea, nongonococcal urethritis
Neurologic	Persistent headache	Central nervous system toxoplasmosis, lymphoma, cryptococcal or TB meningitis, herpes encephalitis
	Memory or concentration deficits	AIDS encephalopathy, chronic meningitis, PML
	Numbness or dysesthesia	AIDS myelopathy, herpes zoster

Note: TB = tuberculosis, MAI = *Mycobacterium avium-intracellulare*, HSV = herpes simplex virus, CMV = cytomegalovirus, PCP = *Pneumocystis carinii* pneumonia, ITP = idiopathic thrombocytopenic purpura, PML = progressive multifocal leukoencephalopathy.

Table 7-3 lists recommended laboratory tests. The following sections address the role of these tests in managing the seropositive, asymptomatic patient.

Table 7-2. Body areas, signs, and possible causes to consider during physical examination in HIV-positive, asymptomatic adults

Area	Sign	Possible causes
Vital signs	Weight loss, fever	
Lymph nodes	Lymphadenopathy	AIDS-related lymphadenopathy, CMV, syphilis, lymphoma, Kaposi's sarcoma, TB
Skin	Scaling lesions	Seborrheic dermatitis, psoriasis
	Vesicle	Herpes simplex, herpes zoster, molluscum contagiosum
	Purpura	ITP
	Violaceous papule, macule, or nodule	Kaposi's sarcoma
Eyes		
Fundoscopic exam	Retinal hemorrhage	CMV retinitis
	Yellow-white retinal infiltrate	CMV or toxoplasma retinitis
Visual field exam	Field defects	CMV or toxoplasma retinitis
Mouth	White plaques	Oral candidiasis, hairy leukoplakia
	Ulcers	HSV, CMV
Chest	Rales	PCP, TB, bacterial pneumonia
Abdominal	Hepatomegaly	Lymphoma, TB, MAI, fungal infection
	Splenomegaly	ITP, lymphoma, fungal infection

(*continued*)

Table 7-2. (*Continued*)

Area	Sign	Possible causes
Anorectal	Ulcerations	HSV, CMV
	Violaceous anal macules or nodules	Kaposi's sarcoma
Genitourinary	Ulcerations	Primary syphilis, chancroid, HSV
	Discharge	Gonorrhea, nongonococcal urethritis
Nervous system	Cognitive deficits	AIDS encephalopathy
	Motor or sensory deficits	AIDS neuropathy or encephalopathy, CNS infections
	Ataxia	CNS toxoplasmosis, lymphoma

Note: CMV = cytomegalovirus, TB = tuberculosis, PCP = *Pneumocystis carinii* pneumonia, CNS = central nervous system, MAI = *Mycobacterium avium-intracellulare*, ITP = idiopathic thrombocytopenic purpura, HSV = herpes simplex virus.

Table 7-3. Recommended laboratory studies and follow-up frequencies for HIV-positive, asymptomatic adults

Study	Frequency of follow-up
T lymphocytes	Every 6 months
CBC	Every year*
Chemistry panel	Every 2–3 years*
Urinalysis	Every 2–3 years*
PPD with anergy battery	Every year (discontinue if anergic)
Chest x-ray	Only if anergic or prior history of positive PPD
Serologic tests for syphilis	Every year*
Hepatitis B serologic tests	Once (preimmunization)
Toxoplasma titers	Once (baseline)

*Recommended frequency when laboratory results are normal; when results are abnormal, tests should be repeated as clinically indicated.

T-lymphocyte studies and other prognostic markers

One of the issues confronting the primary care clinician is whether asymptomatic individuals who are at increased risk of becoming ill can be identified. Cohort studies are accumulating a wealth of data on prognostic markers for progression to AIDS. The most extensive data exist on the interrelated T-lymphocyte studies: the CD4 lymphocyte (also known as the *T4* or *helper lymphocyte*) count, the percentage of total lymphocytes that have the CD4 marker, and the ratio of these cells to those with the CD8 marker (also called the *T8* or *suppressor lymphocyte*). It is not yet clear which of these indices is the most accurate prognostic marker.

Table 7-4 presents data from one of the largest cohort studies, the Multicenter AIDS Cohort Study.[1, 2] These data show a sharp increase in the risk of developing AIDS as CD4 lymphocyte levels or the CD4 : CD8 ratio decrease. Other cohort studies show similar results.[3] The CD4 cell count is the best-studied prognostic marker, but its drawbacks include high cost and lack of precision. Repeat testing may show as much as a 25 percent variation in CD4 cell counts. While large changes in T-lymphocyte data should be considered significant, the clinician must not overinterpret small changes, and must be alert to trends rather than to isolated values.

Beta-2 microglobulin is a protein that is part of the major histocompatibility complex class I antigen. Its serum levels are thought to reflect lymphocyte turnover. Cohort studies show that increased levels of beta-2 microglobulin are correlated with an increased risk of progression to AIDS.[4] This increased risk appears to be independent of CD4 lymphocyte counts. Beta-2 microglobulin is used in other studies of immune function and is thus generally available and relatively inexpensive. However, the prognostic data

Table 7-4. Initial CD4 T-Cell levels and CD4:CD8 ratios in seropositive men and probability of developing AIDS in 18 months

CD4 T cells (no./mm^3)	Probability (%)	CD4:CD8 ratio	Probability (%)
100	58	0.1	69
200	33	0.2	36
300	16	0.4	13
400	8	0.6	6
500	4	0.8	3

Source: Reprinted with permission from Fahey JL, Taylor JM, Korns, E, Nishanian P. Diagnostic and prognostic factors in AIDS. *Mt. Sinai J Med* 1986;53:657–663.

are more limited than are data from CD4 lymphocyte counts, and current trials of antiretroviral therapy in asymptomatic individuals are primarily based on CD4 lymphocyte levels.

Other prognostic markers currently under study include neopterin, a product of macrophages, and p24 antigen, a component of HIV which provides a marker for viral replication. Early data suggest that these markers are also independent predictors for the development of AIDS.[5, 6] Isolation of HIV from plasma also reflects viral replication and is more predictive than are these markers (see Chap. 5). However, HIV cultures are not available to most clinicians.

Thus, we can identify asymptomatic, seropositive individuals at increased risk of developing AIDS. In the near future, data from cohort studies are likely to identify combinations of laboratory markers, symptoms, and physical findings that further improve our ability to predict this risk. The essential question for the clinician, however, is whether this information is useful in managing patients.

Preliminary data suggest that treatment with zidovudine delays or prevents progression to overt AIDS in asymptomatic, HIV-infected persons with CD4 lymphocyte counts less than 500/mm^3 (see Chap. 11). Future studies may result in further expansion of the indications for zidovudine, other antiretroviral drugs, or additional prophylactic measures in asymptomatic individuals, based on prognostic markers. Most physicians initiate prophylaxis for PCP based on T-lymphocyte studies, a practice that is discussed later and in Chap. 8. Physicians may also want to increase the frequency of follow-up visits for patients with low CD4 lymphocyte counts to improve surveillance for opportunistic infections.

We have found prognostic information to be helpful when deciding on diagnostic strategies for nonspecific complaints, such as headaches and respiratory symptoms, which could be due to opportunistic infections. A frequently encountered situation in our clinical practice, for example, is an otherwise asymptomatic, seropositive patient who presents with new onset of a cough, rhinitis, and mild shortness of breath, which have persisted for several days. If the patient has had a T-lymphocyte study within the preceding year which showed that the CD4 : CD8 ratio is greater than 0.8, the prior probability of developing an opportunistic infection is less than 3 percent. This prognostic information often decreases our index of suspicion for an opportunistic infection sufficiently that such a patient can be sent home with careful follow-up. In contrast, for a patient with a CD4 : CD8 ratio less than 0.1, whose risk of developing AIDS within 18 months is nearly 70 percent, a chest x-ray and a blood gas analysis would be indicated, followed by a gallium scan or other tests if the diagnosis remains uncertain.

In summary, we suggest that T-lymphocyte studies be done every 6 months. This marker currently has the largest accumulated data base, and recommendations for interventions such as PCP prophylaxis or zidovudine therapy are largely based on these tests. In the near future, new data may alter this suggestion, and the addition of other markers may be found to be useful.

Complete blood cell count

The complete blood cell count (CBC) may reveal HIV-related anemia, thrombocytopenia, or lymphopenia. In addition to alerting the physician to these conditions, major cohort studies have shown a strong association between these abnormalities and progression to AIDS. As an example, the Multicenter AIDS Cohort Study found that asymptomatic, seropositive individuals with hemoglobin levels less than 13.5 g/dl were nearly 20 times as likely to progress to AIDS over the succeeding 9 months than were individuals with normal hemoglobin levels.[2] Some studies have found that, on multivariate analysis, the value of abnormalities in the CBC to predict progression to AIDS appears to be captured by other variables, such as the T-lymphocyte analysis.[2] However, the CBC is rapid, inexpensive, and easily available, and it may be a useful surrogate for these other tests under certain circumstances.

HIV-infected individuals are susceptible to the same causes of anemia as other patients. Thus, if anemia is detected, an evaluation for treatable causes of this condition is in order. We repeat the CBC yearly if the results are normal.

Blood chemistries

Several tests or chemistry batteries deserve particular attention. Elevated blood urea nitrogen and creatinine levels may indicate the presence of AIDS-related renal disease. Abnormalities of liver enzymes may suggest the early stages of liver infiltration by opportunistic organisms or viral hepatitis. Elevated total protein may be due to the hypergammaglobulinemia found in AIDS, and decreased albumin may indicate poor nutrition due to AIDS-related gastrointestinal disturbances. Because there are few treatment options for most of these conditions, however, the value of these tests is limited. Once an initial evaluation is completed, it is probably useful to repeat chemistry batteries only at 2- to 3-year intervals unless there are symptoms that warrant repeat testing. Some clinicians, however, repeat these tests annually.

Urinalysis

Urinalysis may reveal proteinuria due to AIDS nephropathy. The currently untreatable nature of this complication, however, limits the utility of routine urinalysis.

Tuberculin testing, anergy batteries, and chest x-rays

The incidence of active *Mycobacterium tuberculosis* infection is markedly elevated among HIV-infected patients. The vast majority of cases of tuberculosis represent the reactivation of latent infection due to past exposure rather than the acquisition of new infection.[7] This underlines the importance of tuberculin testing and implies that effective prophylaxis of tuberculosis could prevent most cases of tuberculosis in HIV-infected patients. This practice is discussed later, in the section on disease prophylaxis and in Chap. 8.

The reliability of tuberculin skin testing in HIV-seropositive patients is complicated by the possibility of anergy, which results in a false-negative purified protein derivative (PPD) skin test. If an anergic patient gives a history of a past positive tuberculin skin test, he or she must be treated as if tuberculin positive.

Anergic patients should receive a chest x-ray for evidence of latent tuberculosis. In patients who are not anergic, a chest x-ray is unlikely to reveal treatable, occult pulmonary disease in an asymptomatic patient. The utility of a baseline chest x-ray for comparison months or years later is also of questionable value. For these reasons, we believe that routine chest x-rays are not indicated unless patients are anergic. There has been little careful study of these issues, however.

Screening and management of syphilis

The management of syphilis in HIV-infected persons is complex, poorly studied, and controversial. There is a high incidence of past or present syphilis in most HIV-seropositive populations, and anecdotal reports suggest that syphilis may be more virulent and more difficult to treat in HIV-infected persons.[8] We recommend that all patients have a baseline serologic test for syphilis, including both VDRL (or equivalent screening test) and the fluorescent treponemal antibody-absorbed (FTA-ABS) test (or other *Treponema pallidum*–specific assay). A quantitative VDRL, which probably remains a reliable indicator of syphilis activity even in HIV-infected persons, should be repeated annually in persons with reactive FTA-ABS tests or who continue high-risk sexual behavior.[8]

Recent evidence suggests that, contrary to standard recommendations, single-dose treatment with benzathine penicillin may not be sufficient in HIV-infected individuals even in early stages of syphilis.[9] Although evidence is lacking as to what constitutes adequate therapy, it appears prudent to use at least three weekly doses of 2.4 million units of benzathine penicillin.

Whether HIV-infected individuals with untreated syphilis of all stages should have their cerebrospinal fluid (CSF) examined to guide treatment remains a point of controversy. There is a consensus that individuals with neurologic symptoms or signs, or individuals with latent syphilis of more than 1 year or of unknown duration should have a CSF examination performed.[10] If this is not possible, treatment for presumed neurosyphilis is recommended.

Although the CDC does not currently suggest CSF examination in other stages of syphilis, we believe that CSF examination should be considered in all stages of syphilis in HIV-infected individuals; if spinal fluid is abnormal, neurosyphilis regimens of penicillin should be used. We recognize that serologic tests for syphilis on CSF are insensitive, that CSF leukocytosis and an elevated protein level commonly result from HIV infection itself, and that performance of lumbar punctures may pose logistical and compliance problems in the primary care setting. However, in view of the frequency of central nervous system penetration by *T. pallidum*,[9] and the fact that containment of the organism appears to be a cell-mediated immune function, we feel that erring on the side of overtreatment is justified.[11] Regardless of the treatment regimen chosen, careful follow-up with repeat VDRL or equivalent testing at 1, 2, 3, 6, and 12 months, or until results revert to negative, and repeat CSF assessment if the initial results are abnormal, are essential to determine whether treatment has been effective.

Hepatitis B serology

As discussed later, hepatitis B virus (HBV) vaccination is suggested for HIV-seropositive patients who do not have past exposure to HBV. Whether individuals should be tested for past exposure prior to HBV vaccination is a question of cost effectiveness, as there is no evidence that vaccinating previously exposed individuals is harmful.[12] The prevalence of past exposure to HBV among most HIV-seropositive populations is so high that it is quite cost effective to screen prior to vaccination, and it is therefore suggested that screening be performed as part of the baseline evaluation of HIV-infected patients.[12]

Toxoplasma titers

Among patients with AIDS who have serologic evidence of past exposure to *Toxoplasma gondii,* 6–30 percent may develop toxoplasma encephalitis during the course of the disease.[13, 14] Thus, the finding of a positive

Table 7-5. Recommended prophylactic measures for HIV-seropositive patients

Measure	Recommendation
Vaccination against:	
Influenza	Yearly
Pneumococcus	Once
Hepatitis B	Once (series of three)
Prophylaxis for:	
PCP	If CD4 cell count is less than 200/mm^3 or less than 20 percent of lymphocytes
Tuberculosis	If positive PPD or a history of positive PPD exists

toxoplasma titer should alert the clinician to an increased risk of developing toxoplasmosis of the central nervous system as immunodeficiency progresses.

A titer that shows a significant increase over baseline values during suspected toxoplasmosis constitutes evidence of active infection. Therefore, in the small number of cases in which computerized tomography (CT) fails to reveal lesions when toxoplasmosis is in fact present, serologic testing occasionally may provide valuable information.[13] However, variations in assay methods between laboratories do not allow accurate comparisons of results from one laboratory to another.

PROPHYLACTIC MEASURES

A number of measures (Table 7-5) may help to prevent or delay progression of HIV or may prevent infections that occur frequently in HIV-infected individuals. These measures include the use of zidovudine and other antiviral agents; vaccinations for influenza, pneumococcus, and hepatitis; and prophylaxis for tuberculosis and PCP.

Zidovudine

Recent data suggest that zidovudine may work best as a prophylactic agent when started at an early stage of HIV infection, before a significant amount of viral replication has taken place. Most asymptomatic or mildly symptomatic, HIV-infected persons with CD4 lymphocyte counts less than 500/mm^3 should be treated with zidovudine, 500–800 mg/per day in four to five divided doses (see Chap. 11).

Prophylaxis for PCP

In view of the significant risk of patients with low CD4 lymphocyte counts (e.g., less than 200/mm^3) developing PCP, most physicians view this as an indication for prophylaxis with trimethoprim-sulfamethoxazole, aerosolized pentamidine, or other agents, despite the continuing lack of studies that directly address the risks and benefits of such prophylaxis in asymptomatic individuals. The CDC has recently provided guidelines for prophylaxis against PCP in HIV-infected persons,[15] as discussed in Chap. 8.

Prophylaxis for tuberculosis

All HIV-seropositive, tuberculin-reactive patients should receive isoniazid prophylaxis against active tuberculosis for at least a year.[7, 16] It is unknown whether isoniazid should be continued longer, perhaps indefinitely, for persons with advanced immunodeficiency (see Chap. 8).

Influenza vaccine

Influenza vaccine is recommended annually for all HIV-infected persons for two reasons. First, complications of influenza, such as bacterial pneumonia, which could presumably have increased morbidity in HIV-infected individuals, can be prevented. Second, influenza symptoms can be confused with those of opportunistic infections, so prevention may avoid patient anxiety and expensive, potentially painful diagnostic interventions. In the asymptomatic individual, vaccination response rates have been found to be close to those of the general population.[17, 18] Influenza vaccine appears to be very safe in this population. There has been no in vivo evidence, for example, to support the fear that vaccination might paradoxically stimulate HIV viral replication and accelerate the course of HIV disease.[18]

Pneumococcal vaccine

Pneumococcal vaccine is recommended because of the increased incidence of pneumococcal pneumonia and sepsis among patients with AIDS.[19] The vaccine, administered once, is best given at an early stage of HIV infection, when antibody responses are close to those of the general population.[17]

Hepatitis vaccine

Hepatitis B vaccine is recommended for all HIV-infected individuals who have been found by serologic screening for hepatitis to have had no prior exposure to the virus. One reason is that the same behaviors that predispose a person to HIV disease also place a person at high risk for hepatitis B. Also, HIV-infected individuals are at greater risk than the general population of becoming hepatitis B carriers once they are infected.[20] Vaccination is thus an important means of preventing the spread of hepatitis B. As with the other vaccines recommended, hepatitis B antibody response rates are best when given at an early stage of HIV infection.[21]

PSYCHOLOGICAL AND SOCIAL SUPPORTS

The psychosocial aspects of AIDS are discussed in more detail in Chap. 12. Briefly, in caring for the asymptomatic, seropositive patient, the strengths and weaknesses of the individual's support network, symptoms of depression, and risk of suicide must be assessed. If available, a support group can be suggested. Other means of strengthening support from family and friends may need to be explored. A meeting that includes the patient's partner may be helpful in regard to these issues. Individual counseling may be indicated as well.

PREVENTION OF SPREAD OF HIV

HIV-seropositive, asymptomatic individuals are the major reservoir for the spread of HIV infection. The physician who cares for these individuals is thus in an important position to decrease the transmission of HIV by providing counseling about changing high-risk behaviors. In addition, anxiety about infecting other individuals can have a profound impact on the lives of HIV-infected persons. This anxiety may be ameliorated by discussing issues such as safe sex. For these reasons, counseling about safe sex and, where appropriate, safer drug-use techniques are important aspects of care for the HIV-infected patient. In some states, the physician may be obligated to take steps to ensure that exposed sexual and needle-sharing partners are informed. These issues are discussed in Chaps. 3 and 6.

ENCOURAGING A HEALTHY LIFESTYLE

Stress and poor nutrition may adversely affect the body's immune system.[22] Although there are limited data on the effect of lifestyle on the course of HIV infection, this provides a logical rationale for encouraging HIV-infected patients to pursue a healthy lifestyle. In addition, it is plausible that repeated infections (e.g., STDs) and other immunologic stimuli (e.g., injection of foreign material) can accelerate HIV replication by activating infected lymphocytes or macrophages. Thus, stress reduction, exercise, proper nutrition, maintenance of safe sexual practices, and avoidance of drug use should be emphasized routinely.

CONCLUSIONS

We are coming to view AIDS as the tip of the iceberg of a chronic disease in which most individuals are asymptomatic. We have outlined measures that hold promise for altering the course of HIV infection at this stage, improving quality of life, and decreasing transmission of HIV and other potentially transmissible agents. Until there is a cure for AIDS, much more remains to be learned about what should be done in this stage of HIV infection, and recommendations can be expected to evolve as new evidence accumulates.

Acknowledgment The authors wish to thank Gerald Friedland, M.D., and Abigail Zuger, M.D., for their comments on the manuscript and Clara Jones, M.D., for her input into many of the clinical issues discussed in the chapter.

REFERENCES

1. Fahey JL, Taylor JM, Korns E, Nishanian P. Diagnostic and prognostic factors in AIDS. *Mt Sinai J Med* 1986;53:657–663.

2. Polk BF, Fox R, Brookmeyer R, et al. Predictors of the acquired immunodeficiency syndrome developing in a cohort of seropositive homosexual men. *N Engl J Med* 1987;316:61–66.

3. Goedart JJ, Biggar RJ, Melbye M, et al. Effect of T4 count and cofactors of the incidence of AIDS in homosexual men infected with HIV. *JAMA* 1987;257:331–334.

4. Moss AR, Bacchetti, P, Osmond D, et al. Seropositivity for HIV and the development of AIDS or AIDS-related condition: Three year follow-up of the San Francisco General Hospital cohort. *Br Med J* 1988;296:745–750.

5. Moss AR. Predicting who will progress to AIDS. *Br Med J* 1988;297:1067–1068.

6. Melmed RN, Taylor JMG, Detels R, et al. Serum neopterin changes in HIV-infected subjects: Indicator of significant pathology, CD4 cell changes, and the development of AIDS. *AIDS* 1989;2:70–76.

7. Selwyn PA, Hartel D, Lewis VA, et al. A prospective study of the risk of tuberculosis among intravenous drug users with HIV infection. *N Engl J Med* 1989;320:545–550.

8. Johns DR, Tierney M, Felsenstein D. Alteration in the natural history of neurosyphilis by concurrent infection with the human immunodeficiency virus. *N Engl J Med* 1987;316:1569–1572.

9. Lukehart SA, Hook EW, Baker-Zander SA, et al. Invasion of the central nervous system by *Treponema pallidum:* Implications for diagnosis and treatment. *Ann Intern Med* 1988;109:855–862.

10. Centers for Disease Control. Sexually transmitted diseases treatment guidelines, 1989, *MMWR* 1989 (in press).

11. Tramont EC. Syphilis in the AIDS era. *N Engl J Med* 1987;316:1600–1601.

12. Centers for Disease Control. Recommendations for protection against viral hepatitis. *Ann Intern Med* 1985;103:391–402.

13. Israeski DM, Remington JS. Toxoplasma encephalitis in patients with AIDS. *Infect Dis Clin N Am* 1988;2:429–445.

14. Luft BJ, Brooks RG, Conley FK, et al. Toxoplasmic encephalitis in patients with acquired immune deficiency syndrome. *JAMA* 1984;252:913–917.

15. Centers for Disease Control. Guidelines for prophylaxis against *Pneumocystis carinii* pneumonia for persons infected with human immunodeficiency virus. *MMWR* 1989;38:S1–S9.

16. Centers for Disease Control. Diagnosis and management of mycobacterial infection and disease in persons with human immunodeficiency virus infection. *Ann Intern Med* 1987;106:254–256.

17. Huang K, Ruben FL, Rinaldo CR, et al. Antibody responses after influenza and pneumococcal immunization in HIV-infected homosexual men. *JAMA* 1987;257:2047–2050.

18. Nelson KE, Clements ML, Miotti P, et al. The influence of human immunodeficiency virus (HIV) infection on antibody responses to influenza vaccines. *Ann Intern Med* 1988;109:383–388.

19. Polsky B, Gold JWM, Whimbey E, et al. Bacterial pneumonia in patients with the acquired immunodeficiency syndrome. *Ann Intern Med* 1986;104:38–41.

20. Taylor PE, Stevens CE, Rodriguez de Cordoba S, et al. Hepatitis B virus and human immunodeficiency virus: Possible interactions. In: Zuckerman AJ, ed. *Viral hepatitis and liver disease*. Proceedings of the International Symposium on Viral Hepatitis and Liver Disease, London, May 26–28, 1987. New York: Alan R. Liss, Inc., 1988:198–200.

21. Collier AC, Corey L, Murphy VL, et al. Antibody to human immunodeficiency virus and suboptimal response to hepatitis B vaccination. *Ann Intern Med* 1988;109:101–105.

22. Chlebowski RT. Significance of altered nutritional status in acquired immune deficiency syndrome (AIDS). *Nutr Cancer* 1985;7:85–91.

8

Clinical Manifestations and Approach to Management of HIV Infection and AIDS

Ann C. Collier
Terence C. Gayle
Fredrick H. Bahls

Persons with HIV infection show a broad spectrum of clinical presentations from asymptomatic to life-threatening. Conceptually, clinical issues relate to HIV infection and to complications of HIV-induced immunodeficiency. The number and variety of specific infectious and malignant complications associated with AIDS have increased, but so has information about diagnosis and treatment. Many complications of AIDS are treatable, and treatment may prolong survival and improve the quality of life for affected persons. However, therapy for some complications is suboptimal. Some widely used treatments are experimental, and for other complications, no specific treatment is available. Multiple opportunistic complications frequently coexist, and some require lifelong treatment. However, the principles of care are no different for this problem that for other medical conditions. The management of selected clinical syndromes is discussed in Chap. 9.

CLASSIFICATION OF HIV INFECTION

The CDC introduced the classification scheme most widely used to characterize the spectrum of disorders caused by HIV.[1] Persons infected

The opinions, conclusions, and proposals in this chapter are those of the authors and may not represent the views of the Seattle Veterans Administration Medical Center.

Table 8-1. CDC classification system for HIV infection

Group		Description
I		Acute HIV infection; requires documentation of seroconversion
II		Asymptomatic, seropositive; no current or previous signs or symptoms of infection
III		Persistent generalized lymphadenopathy; palpable lymph nodes at two or more extrainguinal sites
IV		Severe AIDS-related diseases
	A	Constitutional disease; unexplained fever or diarrhea for more than 1 month or loss of more than 10 percent of body weight
	B	Neurologic disease; unexplained dementia, myelopathy, or neuropathy
	C-1	Opportunistic infection; symptomatic or invasive disease due to 1 of the 12 secondary infectious diseases specified in the original CDC surveillance definition for AIDS*
	C-2	Other infections; symptomatic or invasive due to 1 of 6 other specified infectious diseases: oral hairy leukoplakia, multidermatomal herpes zoster virus infection, recurrent *Salmonella* bacteremia, nocardiosis, tuberculosis, or oral candidiasis
	D	Opportunistic malignancies of the CDC surveillance definition: Kaposi's sarcoma, non-Hodgkin's lymphoma, primary central nervous system lymphoma
	E	Other conditions

*PCP, chronic cryptosporidiosis, toxoplasmosis, extraintestinal strongyloidiasis, isosporiasis, candidiasis (esophageal, bronchial, or pulmonary), cryptococcosis, histoplasmosis, mycobacterial infection with *Mycobacterium avium* complex or *M. kansasii*, cytomegalovirus infection, chronic mucocutaneous or disseminated herpes simplex virus infection, and progressive multifocal leukoencephalopathy.

with HIV are grouped into four main categories (Table 8-1). Because the natural history of HIV is incompletely understood, this scheme was not designed to have prognostic significance. Persons are classified into the highest group for which they meet the assignment criteria.

Group I includes individuals with acute HIV infection, which usually occurs 1–12 weeks after exposure. The infection may be asymptomatic; may resemble mononucleosis with malaise, fever, lymphadenopathy, rash, headache, and myalgias or arthralgias; or may result in aseptic meningitis. The symptoms are usually self-limited, and treatment is supportive. Diagnosis of Group I infection requires documentation of HIV antibody seroconversion.

Asymptomatic, HIV-seropositive individuals comprise Group II. Group III includes persons with persistent generalized lymphadenopathy, defined by the presence of lymph nodes measuring at least 1 cm in diameter in at least two extrainguinal areas for at least 3 months. Many persons with persistent generalized lymphadenopathy are asymptomatic, although some have mild constitutional symptoms such as night sweats or fatigue. Group II or III patients may have abnormalities such as leukopenia, lymphopenia, thrombocytopenia, hypergammaglobulinemia, or anemia. Patients with Group II or III infection appear to have equal risk for the subsequent development of overt AIDS.

Group IV disease, which includes AIDS and the entity formerly known as *AIDS-related complex (ARC),* is divided into five subgroups (Table 8-1). Subgroup A includes persons with constitutional symptoms, such as persistent unexplained fever, significant weight loss, or persistent diarrhea without identifiable cause. Although the term *AIDS-related complex* has been widely used to refer to constitutional symptoms and a wasting syndrome associated with HIV, no uniform definition has been established. Before attributing symptoms to HIV infection, other potential causes must be excluded (see Chap. 9). Directed laboratory studies should be based on the patient's symptoms and signs. Even in the absence of identifiable complications, this syndrome may cause extreme debilitation. Current approaches to treatment include nutritional support, treatment with antiviral drugs such as zidovudine, prophylaxis for PCP for patients with depressed CD4 cell counts, specific treatment of any complicating infections, and psychosocial support.

Persons with significant neurologic disease fall into subgroup B of Group IV unless they also have a specific opportunistic disease characteristic of AIDS. Group IV, subgroup C, is itself divided into two categories: C-1 includes persons with 1 or more of the 12 opportunistic infections included in the 1985 CDC surveillance definition of AIDS. C-2 refers to six other infectious diseases, including recurrent *Salmonella* bacteremia and multidermatomal herpes zoster. Subgroup D refers to the malignancies recognized in the present CDC disease surveillance definition, including Kaposi's sarcoma and non-Hodgkin's lymphoma. Subgroup E includes conditions that are not part of other subgroups.

In addition to the CDC system, other classification schemes for HIV have been proposed. The Walter Reed staging classification system, another widely used scheme, assigns infected persons to six categories based on CD4 cell counts, delayed cutaneous hypersensitivity testing, presence or absence of thrush, persistent lymphadenopathy, or opportunistic infections.[2] Details of the staging are shown in Table 8-2. This scheme is based on the

Table 8-2. Walter Reed classification system for HIV infection

Stage*	HIV†	Chronic lymphadenopathy‡	CD4 cells/mm^3	Anergy§	Thrush	OI‖
WR 0#	–	–	>400	None	–	–
WR 1	+	–	>400	None	–	–
WR 2	+	+	>400	None	–	–
WR 3	+	±	<400	None	–	–
WR 4	+	±	<400	Partial	–	–
WR 5	+	±	<400	Complete and/or	+	–
WR 6	+	±	<400	Partial or complete	±	+

*Additional clinical manifestations should be designated by suffixes: B for constitutional symptoms, K for Kaposi's sarcoma, CNS for HIV-induced neurologic disease, N for neoplasm.

†HIV infection documented by antibodies detected on confirmatory testing or virus isolation.

‡Lymph nodes at two or more extrainguinal sites of 1 cm or more in diameter for more than 3 months.

§Anergy is defined by the response to tetanus, trichophyton, mumps, and *Candida* antigens; "none" is response to two or more antigens, "partial" is response to one antigen, and "complete" is no response to any antigen.

‖OI = opportunistic infection.

#Persons at high risk for acquiring HIV.

Source: Adapted from Redfield RR, Wright DC, Tramont EC. The Walter Reed staging classification for HTLV-III/LAV infection. *N Engl J Med* 1986;314:131–132.

role of the CD4 cell as an important target cell for HIV. This system, however, fails to classify all possible combinations of the proposed features.

The signs, symptoms, and associated complications of HIV infection in children are somewhat different from those in adults. The CDC has developed a separate classification scheme to describe the manifestations of pediatric AIDS. The clinical manifestations and management of pediatric AIDS are discussed in Chap. 10.

SYSTEMIC INFECTIONS

Candidiasis

The most common infection in patients with HIV infection, oral candidiasis, frequently precedes other opportunistic infections (Fig. 8-1). Patients usually complain of a sore mouth; clinical signs may range from diffuse erythema to adherent white plaques. Treatment with oral nystatin or topical clotrimazole troches (four to six times per day) is generally effective, but continued suppressive therapy is usually necessary (Table 8-3). The dose for mainte-

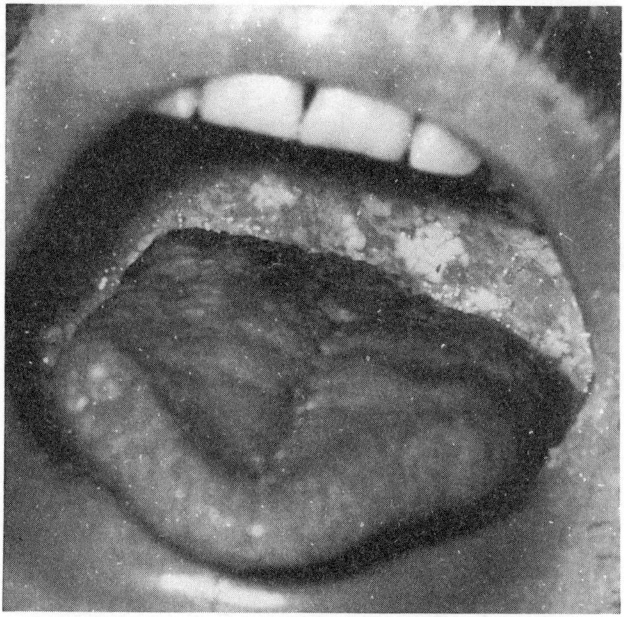

Figure 8-1. Oral candidiasis, showing characteristic adherent white plaques and erythematous mucosa.

nance therapy should be individualized. Ketoconazole (200–400 mg per day) is useful when these regimens are not effective, although decreased gastric acidity in persons with AIDS may prevent absorption of ketoconazole. In addition to ameliorating symptoms, treatment may prevent symptomatic esophageal involvement. For suspected esophagitis, it is important to eliminate other diagnostic possibilities through the use of upper endoscopy, such as infection due to herpes simplex virus or CMV. Low-dose amphotericin B or ketoconazole is used to treat symptomatic esophageal candidiasis (Table 8-3). Severe or recurrent *Candida* vulvovaginitis may occur in women with AIDS. Invasive candidiasis may occur in patients with AIDS but is far less common than in other immunocompromised hosts.

Pneumocystis carinii pneumonia

PCP is the most common serious infection that occurs with AIDS in the United States. Historically, this organism has been classified as a protozoan, but more recently it has been shown to be related to fungi. *P. carinii* is widely distributed, and most persons are exposed to it in childhood. PCP is a typical example of the opportunistic infections that occur with AIDS; reactivation of latent colonization puts immunocompromised hosts at risk for severe pulmonary infection. Symptoms of fever, malaise, nonproductive

Table 8-3. **Treatment of selected opportunistic infections**

Organism	Treatment	Dose	Duration or comments
Candida species			
Oral	Clotrimazole troche *or* Nystatin *or* Ketoconazole	10-mg troche four to six times per day 500,000 units four to six times per day 200–400 mg per day	Until clinically resolved; then taper to maintenance therapy
Esophageal	Ketoconazole *or* Amphotericin B	400 mg per day 0.3 mg/kg per day	Until clinically resolved; use amphotericin B if disease is severe or if no response to oral therapy is obtained; maintenance therapy needed
Cryptococcus neoformans			
Meningitis	Amphotericin B*	0.4–0.6 mg/kg per day *or* 0.8–1.0mg/kg every other day	For 6 weeks or total dose of 1.5–2.0 g followed by lifelong maintenance therapy; optimal dose for maintenance unknown; consider amphotericin B, 100 mg per week, or fluconazole, 100 mg per day
Mycobacterium avium intracellulare	No known effective treatment		

M. tuberculosis	Isoniazid Rifampin Pyrazinamide (PZA)	5 mg/kg per day 9mg/kg per day 25 mg/kg per day	Use three drugs for 2 months, then discontinue PZA; continue two drugs for a minimum of 9 months
Toxoplasma gondii	Pyrimethamine *and* Sulfadiazine *and* Folinic acid	50–100 mg loading dose; then 25–50 mg per day 4 g per day 5 mg per day	For 3–6 months; followed by lifelong maintenance therapy; optimal maintenance dose unknown

Note: Tables 8-3 and 8-4 describe management of PCP; Table 8-5 describes therapy for herpes virus infections.
*Or fluconazole; see text.

cough, and dyspnea may gradually progress over days to weeks, although fulminant respiratory failure also may occur. Chest radiographs typically show diffuse, bilateral, interstitial infiltrates, but findings may be subtle and chest x-rays occasionally may be normal. Because cultures and serologic tests currently are not useful clinically, diagnosis of PCP requires demonstration of organisms in induced sputum, fluid from nasotracheal suction or bronchial-alveolar lavage, or transbronchial biopsy. Monoclonal antibodies to *P. carinii* now exist and have aided in the development of more sensitive and more specific tests to identify the organism in clinical specimens.

Reported mortality for PCP is 10–30 percent. Although early experience with PCP in AIDS suggested mortality rates of 85–90 percent if the pneumonia was severe enough to require ventilatory support, recent experience suggests survival in more than 30 percent of such patients. Several options exist for therapy for PCP, including IV or oral trimethoprim-sulfamethoxazole, IV or aerosol pentamidine, or oral dapsone-trimethoprim (Table 8-4).[3] Therapy is usually given for 14–21 days. IV trimethoprim-sulfamethoxazole, pentamidine, and oral dapsone-trimethoprim appear equally effective, although side effects are common, especially with the first two agents. Minor side effects can often be treated symptomatically with antipyretics, antiemetics, or antihistamines. However, more than 50 percent of patients are unable to tolerate a full course of either of the initial two therapies and require a switch to an alternative regimen. Trimethoprim-sulfamethoxazole has been associated with drug-induced fever, rash, leukopenia, and elevated transaminases. Parenteral pentamidine may cause

Table 8-4. Accepted and investigational treatment regimens for *P. carinii* pneumonia

Accepted*	Investigational
Trimethoprim-sulfamethoxazole 15–20 mg/kg per day of trimethoprim and 75–100 mg/kg per day of sulfamethoxazole every 6 hours (IV or oral); adjust dose to maintain serum trimethoprim level at 5–8 μg/ml	Aerosol pentamidine Trimetrexate and folinic acid Clindamycin and primaquine Dimethyl-fluoro-ornithine
Pentamidine 4 mg/kg per day, given IV by slow infusion over more than 1 hour per dose	
Dapsone and trimethoprim dapsone 100 mg per day (oral) trimethoprim 15–20 mg/kg per day every 6–8 hours (oral)	

*21-day therapy recommended; no benefit for dual regimens.

hypotension, hypoglycemia, hyperglycemia, renal insufficiency, leukopenia, and elevations in liver function test results. It should be given by slow (greater than 1 hour) IV infusion and should not be administered intramuscularly (IM) because it causes sterile abscesses. Dapsone-trimethoprim may cause nausea, vomiting, rash, elevated liver function test results, anemia, and methemoglobinemia; these problems usually do not require discontinuance of treatment. Dapsone should not be used in glucose-6-phosphate dehydrogenase–deficient patients; methemoglobin levels should be monitored during dapsone therapy. If patients are moderately ill or are likely to have malabsorption, therapy should be initiated parenterally. If patients respond well or are stable at diagnosis, oral treatment can be considered. Physicians at centers with experience in managing persons with AIDS frequently diagnose and treat PCP in the outpatient setting. Alternative therapies are under investigation. If patients are intolerant of or are not responding to therapy with conventional agents, trimetrexate should be considered. It is used in conjunction with folinic acid and is available through a treatment investigational new drug protocol (physician's information available at 1-800-537-9978). There appears to be no benefit in the simultaneous use of multiple anti-PCP agents. In addition to antimicrobial therapy, supportive therapy is crucial. The use of corticosteroids for severe PCP is controversial; open trials have suggested utility, but at least one controlled trial has not.

Chemoprophylaxis for PCP in AIDS is indicated for patients who have recovered from an episode of PCP, those with Kaposi's sarcoma who are undergoing chemotherapy, and those with HIV infection who have CD4 cell counts less than 200/mm^3.[4] Comparative trials evaluating several prophylactic regimens are underway, although use of aerosol pentamidine (300 mg per month) is widespread. Using pentamidine as an aerosol creates high levels of the drug in the airways, with little systemic absorption, thereby minimizing systemic toxicity. Local side effects may include cough, irritation of the throat, or wheezing, which are best managed by pretreatment with inhalation of a bronchodilating agent. To maximize deposition in the alveoli, nebulizers used to administer pentamidine should deliver small-diameter particles (0.5–2.5 μM). The major theoretical disadvantage of aerosol pentamidine for PCP prophylaxis is the potential for extrapulmonary pneumocytosis; a small number of cases have been reported, but the prevalence is unclear. In theory, use of systemic antimicrobial agents may provide prophylaxis for other opportunistic infections besides PCP. Other agents in use for PCP prophylaxis include trimethoprim-sulfamethoxazole 3–7 days per week, daily dapsone, parenteral pentamidine one to two times per month, and weekly sulfadoxine-pyrimethamine (Table 8-5). Zidovudine has been shown to decrease the occurrence of opportunistic infections in

Table 8-5. Accepted and investigational regimens for prophylaxis for *Pneumocystis carinii* pneumonia.

Accepted	Investigational
Pentamidine 300 mg per dose every 4 weeks by Respirgard II jet nebulizer (in 6 ml sterile water)	Dapsone Dapsone-trimethoprim Dapsone-pyrimethamine Pyrimethamine-sulfadoxine
Trimethoprim-sulfamethoxazole 160 mg trimethoprim and 800 mg sulfamethoxazole every 12 hours (oral) plus folinic acid 5 mg daily (oral)	Pentamidine (parenteral) Trimethoprim-sulfamethoxazole (three times per week)

patients who have had one episode of PCP, and the drug should be instituted as soon as acute PCP therapy is finished (see Chap. 11 for a discussion of zidovudine).

Mycobacterial infections

The pathogenicity of the atypical mycobacterium *Mycobacterium avium intracellulare* (MAI) in persons with AIDS is controversial, although its high prevalence is not disputed.[5] At least one-third of patients dying with AIDS have disseminated MAI at autopsy. Symptoms attributed to MAI include fever, malaise, weight loss, malabsorption, and diarrhea. Blood cultures are the most useful diagnostic test for detection. MAI is often highly resistant to conventional antituberculous therapy; although a variety of drug combinations have been used for MAI treatment, their utility has not yet been demonstrated. Treatment options include supportive care or a combination of supportive care and a trial of antimicrobial agents. Persons with symptomatic MAI who have adequate hepatic and renal function and who are likely to be compliant with complex regimens may be candidates for an initial 4- to 8-week trial of multiagent antimycobacterial therapy if they desire aggressive treatment. If treatment is undertaken, multiple agents should be used.

Infection with *Mycobacterium tuberculosis* also occurs in persons with HIV infection and may precede other opportunistic infections. All HIV-seropositive persons should have a skin test for evidence of exposure to *M. tuberculosis*. HIV-associated tuberculosis that occurs relatively early in the course of HIV, prior to other opportunistic infections, is usually pulmonary and has a fairly classic clinical presentation. Tuberculosis that occurs in association with advanced HIV infection often presents as nonapical pulmonary disease or at extrapulmonary sites, including lymph nodes, bone marrow, central nervous system, liver, and urinary tract. Therapy for tuberculosis follows standard guidelines, although there is limited experience with short-course chemotherapy for HIV-infected patients, and some experts recommend lifelong isoniazid after therapy is completed (Table 8-3). Response to therapy is good. In contrast to treatment, guidelines for tuberculosis chemoprophylaxis for HIV-infected persons are different than for noninfected persons. Regardless of age, tuberculin skin test–positive persons with HIV should receive chemoprophylaxis. The optimal duration of chemoprophylaxis with isoniazid in HIV infection is unknown, but the need for careful surveillance after either prophylaxis or treatment is clear.

Bacterial infections

Bacterial infections occur in persons with HIV-associated immunosuppression, especially among those with predisposing causes such as IV drug use or indwelling catheters. Data suggest that infective endocarditis may occur more commonly in HIV-infected than in non-HIV-infected drug users. Encapsulated organisms, including *Streptococcus pneumoniae* and *Hemophilus influenzae,* may cause pneumonia or bacteremia in HIV-infected persons. Treatment follows standard guidelines. The incidence of salmonellosis is 20-fold higher in persons with AIDS than in those without AIDS, and recurrent infection is common unless suppressive therapy is used. Other recurrent bacterial infections are particularly problematic in children but may occur in adults as well; treatment with chronic antibacterial agents may be warranted for selected patients. The effects of coexistent HIV infection on syphilis have been controversial; case reports suggest that syphilis serologic tests may be less reliable in some patients with advanced AIDS, that disease manifestations may be altered, and that the response to treatment may be less reliable (see Chap. 7). Other common bacterial complications of HIV include sinusitis, necrotizing gingivitis, and superficial skin infections.

Opportunistic viral infections

Various viral infections are associated with AIDS, including several members of the herpes family. Reactivation of varicella-zoster virus in HIV-seropositive persons suggests immunologic impairment and may precede more serious conditions. Herpes simplex virus may cause persistent ulcerations in the genital or perirectal areas or elsewhere in patients with AIDS or HIV infection. Serologic evidence of Epstein-Barr virus (EBV) and human herpesvirus 6 is common in patients with HIV, but the clinical manifestations of these viruses are less clear than are those of the other herpesviruses. One clinical entity closely associated with EBV is oral hairy leukoplakia, which presents as painless, filiform, "hairy" white or gray lesions on the lateral or inferior sides of the tongue (Fig. 8-2). Diagnosis is usually clinical, including failure to resolve with anticandidal therapy, although this lesion requires biopsy to be definitively identified. Although reported to respond to high-dose acyclovir, oral hairy leukoplakia is usually not treated because it is asymptomatic. However, acyclovir is a widely used, effective antiviral treatment for varicella-zoster virus in compromised hosts and for therapy and prophylaxis of herpes simplex virus (Table 8-6). The occurrence of acyclovir-resistant mutants of herpes simplex virus has been reported in patients with AIDS; the use of vidarabine or the investigational agent foscarnet (trisodium phosphonoformate hexahydrate) is under study.

Of the viral infections commonly associated with AIDS, CMV is the most common etiologic agent and causes the most devastating clinical problem, blindness.[6] Asymptomatic infection is common but the virus may disseminate, leading to involvement of various organs, including the eye, liver, adrenal glands, lung, or brain. CMV retinitis can lead to blindness in one or both eyes and is characterized by progressive retinal inflammation with hemorrhages and exudates (Fig. 8-3). Clinical deterioration can occur over days to weeks, so early diagnosis and intervention are critical. Uncontrolled studies with ganciclovir (dihydroxy-propyl-methyl-guanine,

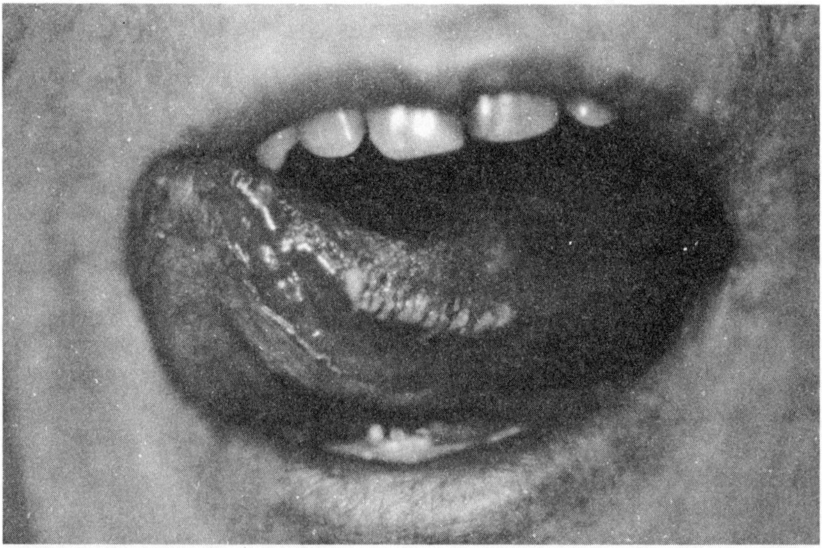

Figure 8-2. Oral hairy leukoplakia, showing characteristic filiform lesions on the lateral tongue border.

Table 8-6. Regimens for herpes group virus infections

Virus	Treatment	Dose	Route
Herpes simplex*	Acyclovir		
Treatment		400 mg every 8 hours	PO
		or	
		5 mg/kg every 8 hours	IV
Prophylaxis		200–400 mg every 8 hours	PO
Varicella-zoster	Acyclovir	10 mg/kg every 8 hours	IV
CMV	Ganciclovir	5 mg/kg every 12 hours; then 5 mg/kg per day†	IV

Note: Some regimens are not approved by the FDA for this indication.
*Genital or mucocutaneous presentations.
†14-day induction regimen followed by daily maintenance.

DHPG) suggest stabilization of vision in two-thirds of those treated. The utility of ganciclovir for CMV pneumonia or gastrointestinal disease is less clear. At present, ganciclovir is available only for parenteral use. Therapy is usually initiated with 5 mg/kg every 12 hours for 14 days (Table 8-6). If tolerated, daily maintenance therapy should be given IV five to seven times a week to prevent relapse. The major side effects of ganciclovir are neutropenia, thrombocytopenia, skin rash, gastrointestinal symptoms, and decreased spermatogenesis. Because of the need for long-term parenteral therapy, patients receiving ganciclovir require indwelling central catheters. To minimize complications, scrupulous catheter care is required. Most patients or their families administer the therapy at home, with assistance of visiting nurses. Serial CBCs are essential for monitoring potential toxicity. Concurrent ganciclovir and zidovudine therapy is poorly tolerated because of the high incidence of neutropenia and is not recommended. Studies of adjuvants such as granulocyte-macrophage colony-stimulating factor (GM-CSF) and alternative anti-CMV drugs, including foscarnet, are underway. Ganciclovir-resistant mutants of CMV have been described, but their prevalence is unknown.

OPPORTUNISTIC MALIGNANCIES

The most common malignant disease associated with AIDS is Kaposi's sarcoma, which is far more common among homosexual than among heterosexual men.[7] Its cause is not known. Cutaneous involvement is almost

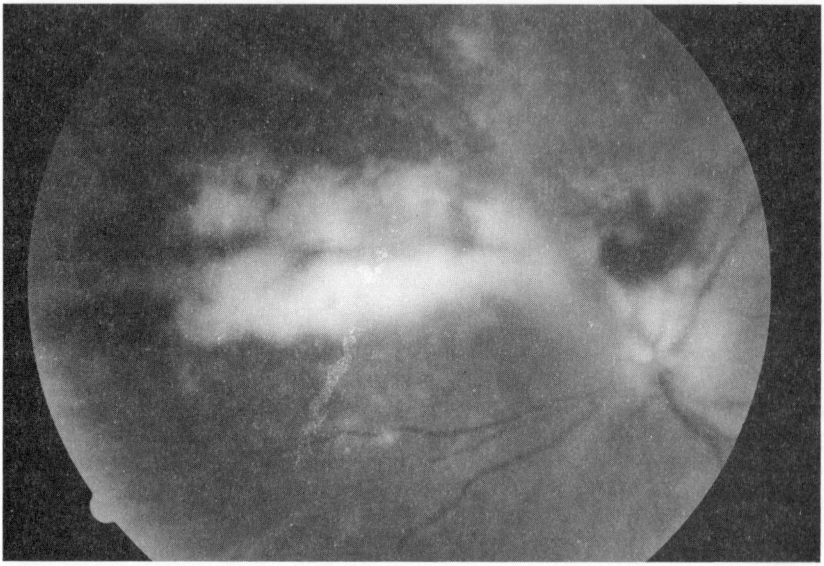

Figure 8-3. Retina, showing characteristic findings of hemorrhage and white retinal necrosis seen with CMV retinitis. (Photograph by Dr. James L. Kinyoun.)

universal in Kaposi's sarcoma (Fig. 8-4), and gastrointestinal involvement, including the mouth, is common. Kaposi's sarcoma lesions may be erythematous, violaceous, black, or multicolored; yellow halos around lesions are common. Lesions may be macular, papular, or nodular and usually are asymptomatic. Because early lesions may be difficult to distinguish from traumatic bruises, careful observation of suspected lesions may be indicated for a few weeks prior to biopsy. Therapeutic approaches include observation, alpha-interferon, single or multiagent chemotherapy, and local irradiation. Persons rarely die of Kaposi's sarcoma itself, but eventually they are likely to develop other opportunistic infections. Zidovudine has no specific activity against Kaposi's sarcoma but appears useful in conjunction with alpha-interferon, although the tolerable doses of each are lower when given simultaneously than when given alone. Other malignancies, including non-Hodgkin's lymphoma and Hodgkin's disease, occur in HIV-infected persons. Although not histologically different, AIDS-associated lymphomas tend to have extranodal presentations. In addition, central nervous system presentations of non-Hodgkin's lymphoma are much more common; mean survival, even with therapy, is measured in months.

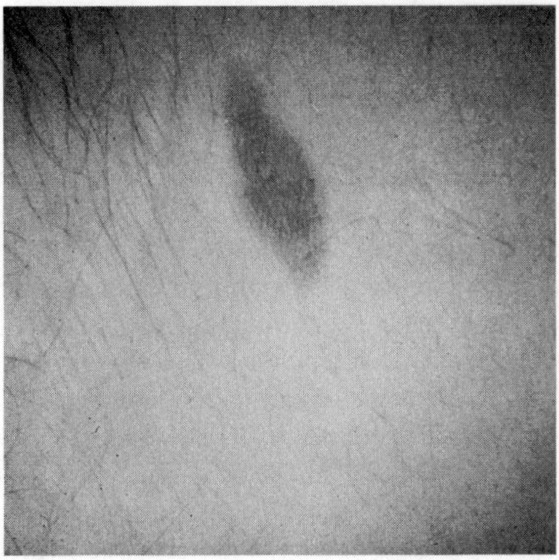

Figure 8-4. Cutaneous Kaposi's sarcoma, showing an early lesion of a nontender, solitary, erythematous macule.

HEMATOLOGIC COMPLICATIONS

A variety of hematologic abnormalities are associated with HIV infection, including autoimmune thrombocytopenia, lymphopenia, neutropenia, anemia, and circulating coagulation inhibitors. Platelet counts may range from near normal to a few thousand. Clinical presentations associated with severe thrombocytopenia are similar to those seen in other patient populations, with easy bruising and petechiae being more common than epistaxis, or gingival or gastrointestinal bleeding. The postulated mechanisms of HIV-associated thromboyctopenia include deposition of immune complexes and complement on platelet membranes or antiplatelet antibodies.

In the past, treatment options for thrombocytopenia included steroids, vincristine, danazol, and splenectomy. More recent data suggest that IV immunoglobulin (with or without steroids) may be useful for treatment of severe thrombocytopenia and that zidovudine is useful for mild to moderate thrombocytopenia.

Lymphopenia is extremely common, because certain subtypes of lymphocytes are the target cells infected by HIV. Neutropenia in patients with AIDS is usually a complication of antimicrobial therapy, including therapy with zidovudine, ganciclovir, trimethoprim-sulfamethoxazole, pentamidine, or pyrimethamine. Although folinic acid is commonly used to prevent cytopenias associated with folate antagonists, little data are available to define its utility in this patient population. Less commonly, neutropenia occurs in HIV-infected persons not being treated with marrow-suppressive agents and may be secondary to the effects of HIV or opportunistic infections on cell production.

The cause of anemia in AIDS may be multifactorial; blood loss and accelerated red blood cell (RBC) destruction may occur but are less common than is decreased RBC production. Because malabsorption, poor appetite, and low caloric intake can contribute to iron or vitamin deficiencies, evaluation of iron stores, vitamin B12, and folate levels is indicated. Suppression of RBC production and development of a moderate normochromic, normocytic anemia is frequent, even in the absence of identifiable opportunistic infections or malignancy. Disseminated MAI is frequently associated with severe anemia. Management of anemia includes systematic evaluation of potential causes, transfusions for symptomatic anemia, and erythropoetin if patients have endogenous erythropoetin levels less than 500 mU/ml. (See Chap. 11 for a discussion of zidovudine-associated anemia.) The lupus anticoagulant, which has been described in AIDS, is usually associated with opportunistic infections but not with bleeding.

NEUROLOGIC COMPLICATIONS

Although AIDS was recognized as a clinical entity in 1981, the extent and variety of neurologic involvement were not appreciated immediately. Clinical involvement of the nervous system occurs in at least 40 percent of patients with AIDS and may be the initial manifestation of HIV infection in 10–30 percent of patients. Several neuropathologic studies of patients with AIDS have found evidence of central nervous system disease in as many as 90 percent of cases. The discrepancy between clinical and pathologic estimates of central nervous system involvement is probably due to subclinical nervous system disease and to the failure to recognize subtle signs of nervous system involvement in patients with devastating systemic disease.

HIV infection can result in a broad spectrum of neurologic disease. No currently recognized characteristics of patients with asymptomatic HIV infection predict the subsequent occurrence of neurologic disease or its nature. We will discuss the most common neurologic presentations associated with HIV infection and emphasize those conditions for which specific therapy is available.

AIDS dementia complex

The most common neurologic presentation of patients with HIV infection is progressive dementia, which has been called the *AIDS dementia complex* or

HIV-associated encephalopathy, and was previously referred to as *subacute encephalitis* or *subacute encephalopathy.*[8] Although this syndrome occurs most commonly after diagnosis of overt AIDS, it may also be the first sign of HIV infection. In persons with AIDS dementia complex, in vitro immunologic studies often show only mild to moderate impairment. The onset of symptoms is usually insidious, but occasionally these patients may present with a fulminant course over days. The untreated full-blown form of this syndrome carries a grave prognosis, with a mean survival of approximately 6 months. Early signs and symptoms in patients with this syndrome can be extremely subtle (Table 8-7), especially in well-educated individuals. In later stages, patients become demented, and the majority have other neurologic signs. The most common finding by computerized tomography (CT) or magnetic resonance (MR) imaging is cortical atrophy. Cerebrospinal fluid studies commonly reveal a mild to moderate increase in protein and, sometimes, a mild mononuclear pleocytosis. Neuropathologic abnormalities occur predominantly in the white matter and subcortical structures, with sparing of the cerebral cortex. Diffuse pallor of the white matter is the most characteristic finding, with clusters of foamy macrophages and multinucleated giant cells present in severe cases.

Table 8-7. Neurologic signs and symptoms of AIDS dementia complex

Cognitive	Motor	Behavioral	Other
	Early		
Forgetfulness	Decreased balance	Apathy	Headache
Decreased concentration	Lower extremity weakness	Social withdrawal	Seizures
Comprehension difficulties	Handwriting changes		Depression
	Late		
Dementia	Psychomotor retardation	Indifference	Organic psychosis
Confusion	Ataxia	Awake	Tremor
Memory loss	Increased tone	Wide-eyed stare	Frontal release signs
	Weakness	Incontinence	

Note: Patients with AIDS dementia complex may present with cognitive (66 percent), motor (45 percent), behavioral (39 percent), or other (20 percent) signs and symptoms of neurologic disorder.

Source: Adapted from Naria BA, Jordan BD, Price RW. The AIDS dementia complex: I. Clinical features. *Ann Neurol* 1986;19:517–524.

Although the cause of this syndrome is not yet known, isolation of HIV from the brains of affected patients, the demonstration of antibodies to HIV in CSF, and clinical improvement with antiviral therapy suggest that the AIDS dementia complex is due to infection of the brain by HIV. One theory is that HIV proteins may cause an immunopathologic or toxic response in the brain. HIV appears to infect primarily microglia and macrophages rather than neurons or astroglia. No definitive treatment for this syndrome has been found, although several reports suggest that zidovudine may be of benefit. The optimal dose of zidovudine for this condition is unclear, but antiviral treatment is indicated (see Chap. 11 and below). It is important to emphasize that patients with other causes of central nervous system involvement may present in precisely the same manner (see below) and that diagnosis of the AIDS dementia complex remains one of exclusion.

Mass lesions

Another common neurologic presentation of patients with HIV infection is an intracerebral mass lesion. Such patients may have headache, focal or generalized seizures, focal weakness, or encephalopathy. On examination, they may have papilledema, hemiparesis, hemisensory loss, aphasia, or mental status abnormalities. CT and MR scanning both can detect the presence of a mass lesion in such patients, but MR may be more sensitive (Figure 8-5*a,b*). However, the exact cause of a mass lesion can be determined only by brain biopsy, because no particular etiologic agent has either a pathognomonic clinical presentation or a neuroradiologic appearance. Similarly, although lumbar puncture should be performed in all patients in whom CT or MR scanning does not show a significant mass, CSF studies often are not specific for a given cause.

The most common cause of central nervous system mass lesions in patients with HIV infection is toxoplasmosis (Fig. 8-6). IgG antibody titer increases or IgM antibodies are not usually detectable in patients with AIDS and toxoplasmosis. It is reasonable in most cases to begin empiric treatment with sulfadiazine and pyrimethamine, especially in patients with detectable antitoxoplasmosis antibody (IgG) (Table 8-3). Patients with toxoplasmosis generally show both clinical and radiologic improvement 1–2 weeks after therapy begins. Therapy in patients who improve needs to be lifelong unless severe side effects develop. After 3–6 months, the doses can probably be decreased if patients are clinically stable. Those patients who are unable to tolerate sulfadiazine may respond to pyrimethamine alone or to therapy with clindamycin, although there are few data on its efficacy. Other agents are under investigation.

Patients with mass lesions in the central nervous system who fail to respond to empiric therapy for toxoplasmosis should be considered for brain

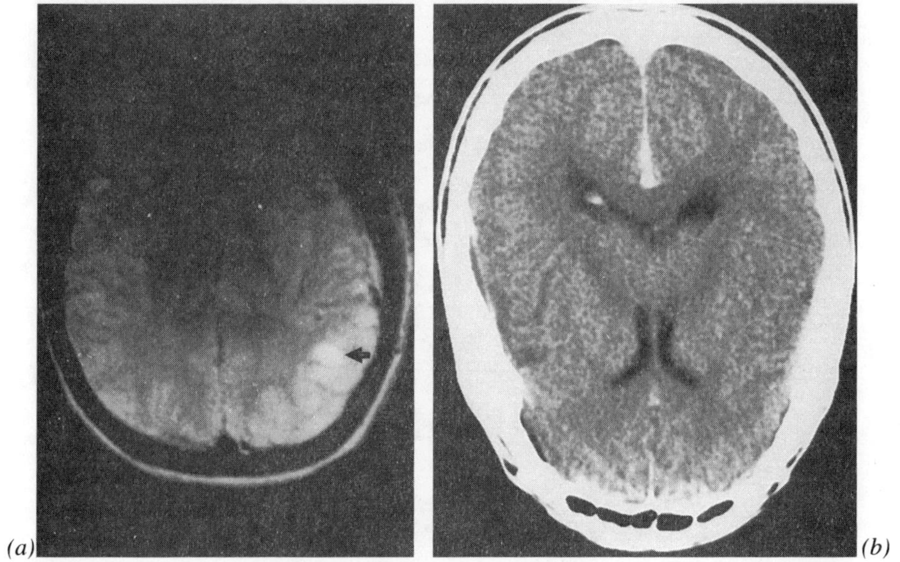

Figure 8-5. (*a*) MR image of the brain of a patient with progressive ataxia, paresthesias, and mental status changes. This cut shows one of multiple lesions present. (*b*) A CT scan taken at the same time was normal. The lesion was visible on a repeat CT scan performed 1 month later. This case demonstrates that MR may detect lesions not apparent on CT scan.

biopsy if the lesion is accessible. An MR scan may reveal additional, more accessible lesions in those patients whose CT scans reveal only a deep lesion. Primary central nervous system lymphoma is the second most common cause of mass lesions in patients with AIDS; a common presenting feature is cranial polyneuropathy. Diagnosis is made by biopsy or, more commonly, at postmortem examination. Because the diagnosis often is postmortem, there is little information on the best therapy. A few patients have shown some response to whole brain irradiation.

Other, less common causes of mass lesions in patients with AIDS include atypical mycobacteria, *M. tuberculosis, Cryptococcus neoformans, Candida,* and progressive multifocal leukoencephalopathy. It is not uncommon for patients to have multiple central nervous system complications, and new diagnoses should be considered if new symptoms appear.

Meningitis

Meningitis is another neurologic presentation of patients with HIV infection. *C. neoformans* is the most frequently identified opportunist causing meningitis in this population. Symptoms may include fever, headache, encephalo-

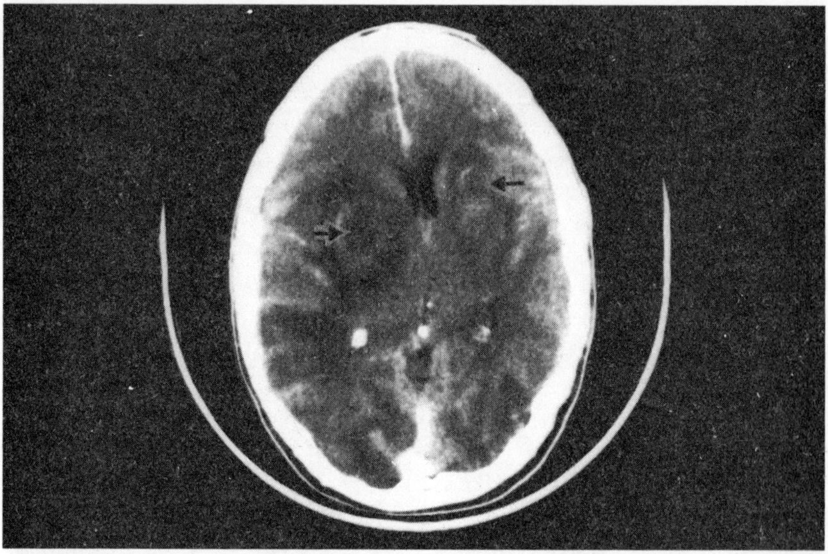

Figure 8-6. This patient presented with focal seizures and left-sided weakness. A CT scan revealed multiple enhancing mass lesions which, on postmortem examination, were shown to be abscesses caused by toxoplasmosis. Other causes of central nervous system mass lesions may have an identical appearance on CT scan.

pathy, or seizures. Patients often have no meningismus. Diagnosis is made by finding elevated levels of cryptococcal antigen in the cerebrospinal fluid, a positive India ink preparation, or fungi upon cerebrospinal fluid culture. Cryptococcal meningitis is usually treated initially with amphotericin B (0.4–0.5 mg/kg per day or twice this dose given on alternate days) (Table 8-3). 5-flucytosine is rarely tolerated. Fluconazole, a triazol agent, appears promising as oral treatment for cryptococcal meningitis, especially for maintenance therapy after a patient has stabilized. Like patients with toxoplasmosis, those with cryptococcal infection need chronic therapy to prevent relapse. The optimal doses and frequency are unknown, but maintenance amphotericin B therapy of 100 mg per week prevented relapse in one study.

Aseptic meningitis is also seen in patients with HIV infection. It may occur during primary infection with HIV or in patients who have no other manifestations of HIV infection. Patients may have headache, fever, meningeal signs, cranial nerve involvement (usually the fifth, seventh, and eighth cranial nerves), and long tract signs such as hyperreflexia. Examination of CSF reveals mononuclear pleocytosis, elevated protein, or increased opening pressure. HIV is believed to be the cause of this syndrome. In most patients the illness is self-limited, although cases with chronic or relapsing features have been reported. Management consists of supportive therapy; anti-HIV therapy should be considered for chronic cases.

Spinal cord syndromes

Several types of spinal cord involvement are associated with HIV infection, the most common being vacuolar myelopathy. Patients develop progressive paraparesis, spasticity, ataxia, incontinence, and extensor plantar responses. Patients frequently also have AIDS dementia complex. Myelography and CSF examination are normal. Pathologically, white matter vacuolation and demyelination are present, most prominently in the dorsal and lateral (corticospinal tract) columns. The cause is unknown, but the frequent association with AIDS dementia complex suggests direct infection of the spinal cord with HIV. Although definitive studies have not been performed, a trial of anti-HIV therapy is appropriate.

Another type of spinal cord involvement is transverse or ascending myelitis. Patients have back pain, usually in the thoracic region; flaccid paresis below the level of the lesion; a sensory level; hyporeflexia; and a neurogenic bladder. They may progress to quadriparesis with cranial nerve involvement. Myelography is normal. CSF may be normal or show lymphocytic pleocytosis. Both CMV and herpes simplex type 2 have been recovered from the spinal cords of such patients, although the yield in CSF is unknown. Because cord compression from epidural abscess or metastatic tumor also can occur in patients with HIV infection, myelography is mandatory in all patients who show evidence of spinal cord involvement.

Peripheral neuropathy

Peripheral neuropathies are a common complication of HIV infection and occur in 10–50 percent of patients. During early stages of HIV infection (CDC Groups I–III, Table 8-1), acute or chronic demyelinating neuropathy may occur. The neuropathy may resemble either the Guillan-Barré syndrome or chronic inflammatory demyelinating polyneuropathy which is seen in non-HIV-infected patients. The only distinguishing feature of the HIV-associated syndromes is the presence of lymphocytic pleocytosis in the CSF. Most patients with inflammatory peripheral neuropathy have fever and malaise. The CSF IgG index is increased, and nerve biopsy shows inflammatory changes. The course is usually benign, with spontaneous remission. Plasmapheresis may benefit patients with a prolonged course.

In patients with overt AIDS, a distal symmetric polyneuropathy is the most common peripheral neuropathy. These patients have painful dysesthesias that may be incapacitating and symmetric sensory loss that rarely includes motor involvement. Diagnostic studies usually are unrevealing, and no clear cause has been determined. Diphenylhydantoin, carbamazepine, or one of the tricyclic antidepressants may benefit patients with severe neuropathic pain.

Myopathy

Several types of myopathy have been described in HIV infection. A common type is a polymyositis-like presentation, with myalgias, proximal muscle weakness, muscle wasting, and elevated creatine phosphokinase. Electromyography shows findings consistent with myopathy, and muscle biopsies may show inflammatory infiltrates. Whether the benefits of steroids for this condition outweigh their immunosuppressive risk is unclear. Myopathy has been described in association with long-term zidovudine therapy, although its frequency, natural history, and best treatment are undetermined. The syndrome is characterized by myalgias and muscle tenderness, weakness, and atrophy that is more prominent in proximal muscles, especially in the buttocks and lower extremities. Initial management of mild symptoms may include observation and continuation of zidovudine and nonsteroidal anti-inflammatory agents; severe involvement merits discontinuance of zidovudine.

Neurologic summary

HIV infection should be considered in any patient with an unusual neurologic disorder. Such patients should undergo evaluation that includes a neuroradiologic examination (CT or MR) and CSF examination. Myelography, brain biopsy, or muscle biopsy is warranted in certain cases. It is important to recognize that patients often may have more than one type of neurologic involvement and require frequent reassessment.

NEUROPSYCHIATRIC MANIFESTATIONS OF HIV INFECTION

There is growing recognition of the wide variety of organic mental disorders associated with HIV infection and AIDS.[9] These neuropsychiatric disorders range from subtle personality changes to severe dementia. Delirium is the most frequent acute organic mental disorder seen in patients with AIDS. It begins abruptly (usually over hours to days) and is characterized by clouded consciousness and disorientation that fluctuate over the course of a day. Delirium is also associated with incoherent speech, altered sleep-wake pattern, perceptual disturbances such as hallucinations, and increased or decreased psychomotor activity. Delirium most often is due to underlying systemic or central nervous system diseases and can result from drug toxicity. Because the underlying conditions are often treatable, it is important to conduct a thorough medical evaluation of any patient with an emerging delirium.

The AIDS dementia complex is the chronic organic mental disorder seen most often in patients with HIV infection.[8] Because cognitive dysfunction can frighten patients, it is important not to overlook the early, subtle symptoms of dementia or to attribute them solely to the emotional reaction to a diagnosis of HIV infection or AIDS. About one-third of patients show increasing apathy and social withdrawal that may mimic major depression. These "negative" symptoms often do not respond to standard antidepressant medications. Other symptoms that should arouse suspicion of early dementia include sleep changes (particularly hypersomnia), impaired judgment, avoidance of complex tasks, increased reliance on lists, obsessive rumination, decreased coordination, handwriting changes, and increased sensitivity to alcohol and prescribed medications. It is not unusual to see presentations of dementia with an overlying (and reversible) delirium.

As many as 80 percent of patients with AIDS without documented neurologic complications show subclinical cognitive impairment upon formal neuropsychological testing. Preliminary research suggests that cognitive dysfunction may occur in a subset of patients in early stages of HIV infection. Because cognitive difficulties may be overlooked by a cursory mental status exam that relies upon orientation questions only, it is crucial that patients with HIV undergo initial assessment with a more thorough exam.

The Mini-Mental State Exam (Table 8-8) is a useful screening test that can be administered at the bedside or in the office in 10–15 minutes.[10] The initial mental status can serve as a baseline for comparison with subsequent examinations. By itself it is not a comprehensive screen of cognitive function or dementia, but it is a test for more gross dysfunction. For example, patients may legitimately complain of memory problems, yet still score in the normal range of 24 or greater. For valid results, persons must have more than an eighth-grade education and no significant sensory or motor deficits—such as cognitive impaired vision (e.g., CMV retinitis) or upper arm weakness—that might interfere with completion of some questions.

Referral for formal neuropsychologic testing is helpful to detect milder cognitive impairment or to document impairment in order to establish the diagnosis of AIDS (CDC Class IV-B) when opportunistic infections and malignancies are absent. Less severe impairment may not constitute global dementia but may interfere with a patient's ability to perform complex tasks. The pattern of impairment seen in AIDS dementia complex resembles that seen in subcortical dementias (e.g., Huntington's disease or progressive supranuclear palsy) more than that in cortical dementias such as Alzheimer's disease. The deficits associated with subcortical dementias include forgetfulness, psychomotor slowing, impaired attention, visuospatial impairment, apathy, and depression. Patients can still learn new material, but they need cues to help retrieve the information. By contrast, in cortical

Table 8-8. Mini-mental state examination

Parameter	Maximum score	Score
Orientation	10	
What is the (year), (season), (day of month), (month), (day of week)? (1 point for each)		—
Where are we: (state), (county), (town), (hospital), (floor)? (1 point for each)		—
Registration	3	
Name three objects: 1 second to say each. Then ask the patient all three after you have said them. Give 1 point for each correct answer. Then repeat them until he learns all three. Count trials and record.		—
Attention and calculation	5	
Serials 7s. 1 point for each correct. Stop after five answers. Alternatively, spell "world" backwards.		—
Recall	3	
Ask for the three objects repeated above. Give 1 point for each correct.		—
Language	9	
Name a pencil and a watch (2 points).		—
Repeat the following: "No ifs, ands, or buts" (1 point)		—
Follow a three-stage command: "Take a paper in your hand, fold it in half, and put it on the floor." (3 points)		—
Read and obey the following:		
"Close your eyes." (1 point)		—
"Write a sentence." (1 point)		—
"Copy this design." (1 point) 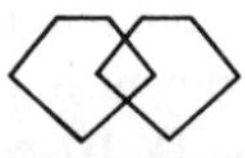		—

Note: Total score possible = 30. Scoring: 24–30 = normal, 20–23 = mild dementia, 10–19 = moderate dementia, below 10 = severe dementia.

Source: Adapted from Folstein MF, Folstein SE, McHugh PR. "mini-mental State"—A practical method for grading the cognitive state of patients for the clinician. *J Psych Res* 1975;12:189–198.

dementias, amnesia, aphasia, apraxia, and agnosia are prominent. Thus, specific assessment of memory, attention, language, reaction time, and visuospatial functions is appropriate when considering a diagnosis of AIDS dementia complex. A briefer set of tests can be given (30–45 minutes) if a patient lacks the stamina to undergo a more comprehensive (3- to 4-hour) neuropsychologic assessment.

As AIDS dementia complex progresses, psychotic features including hallucinations, delusions, and agitated behavior may appear. Occasionally, an acute psychotic episode may herald the onset of the dementia. This is best treated with low doses of high-potency neuroleptics, such as haloperidol or thiothixene with or without the addition of lorazepam (Table 8-9). Patients with AIDS appear to be more sensitive to some extrapyramidal side effects of neuroleptics, such as acute dystonic reactions, akathisia, and bradykinesia. In addition to reducing the neuroleptic dose, the clinician can use amantadine to treat extrapyramidal side effects, rather than more anticholinergic medications such as benztropine. The clinician should also consider other causes of psychoses, such as delirium, drug use and alcohol abuse, or their withdrawal states. Other management strategies for AIDS dementia complex include schemes to help people remember appointments, medication schedules, or reality orientation aids such as calendars, clocks, and familiar attendants.

Other psychiatric presentations have been noted in patients with AIDS and ARC. These include organic mood syndromes (depression and mania) and atypical psychoses. These psychiatric syndromes can develop rapidly in individuals who have neither a premorbid psychiatric history nor a family history of psychiatric disorders. HIV has been implicated as a probable etiologic factor, although other systemic and central nervous system diseases can produce these conditions.

Major depression associated with serious medical illness such as HIV infection or AIDS can be treated with antidepressant medications. As has been observed in major depression associated with cancer, some patients with AIDS will respond to tricyclic antidepressants in lower than usual therapeutic doses. Antidepressant medications that are less anticholinergic, such as desipramine, fluoxetine, or bupropion (all useful for anergic depression), as well as nortriptyline or trazodone (both useful for depression with insomnia), should be used to avoid central anticholinergic toxicity (Table 8-9). Some patients complain about daytime sedation associated with trazodone. Fluoxetine (20 mg each morning, increased to 20 mg twice in the morning after 4 weeks, if necessary) is proving to be useful in treating anergic depression. However, the side effects of nausea and insomnia may limit the utility of this new drug in some patients who already suffer from nausea or insomnia due to other causes. In many cases, the nausea associated with fluoxetine diminishes after the first or second week of use and can be reduced by administering it with food. Bupropion is another new antidepressant now available in the United States which has few anticholinergic

Table 8-9. Treatment regimens for psychiatric disorders in AIDS

Disorder	Drug	Initial dose	Daily dose range	Comments
Major depression (prominent anergy)	Desipramine *or*	10 mg per day	20–300mg	Give in the morning to avoid insomnia unless it causes sedation
	Fluoxetine *or*	20 mg per day	20–60 mg	Give with food Give in the morning to avoid insomnia
	Bupropion	75 mg twice daily	150–300 mg (75–100 mg three times a day)	Use divided doses; no single dose should exceed 150 mg; seizures are a contraindication
Major depression (prominent insomnia)	Nortriptyline *or*	10 mg per day	20–150 mg	Increase by 10-mg increments
	Trazodone	5 mg per day	50–600 mg	May cause priapism in men
Depression (with cognitive impairment)	Methylphenidate	5 mg 3 times in the morning	20–90mg	May increase 10–15 mg per day
Mania or hypomania	Lithium carbonate *or*	300 mg twice daily	600–1200 mg	Monitor thyroid function tests, sodium, creatinine; therapeutic level 0.5–1.2 mEq/L
	Clonazepam *or*	0.5 mg per day	0.5–3.0 mg	Monitor for excessive sedation
	Carbamazepine	200 mg per day	400–2200 mg	Therapeutic level 6–12 μg/dl

Acute psychosis	Haloperidol *or*	0.5–1 mg twice daily	0.5–20 mg	Can be changed to one dose at bedtime after initial week of therapy
	Thiothixene *or*	1–2 mg twice daily	1–30 mg	Can be changed to one dose at bedtime after initial week of therapy
	Perphenazine	4 mg twice daily	4–64 mg	Can be changed to one dose at bedtime after initial week of therapy

and antiadrenergic side effects. Patients should be started on 75 mg twice a day, and the dose can be increased gradually to 100 mg twice a day over 1–2 weeks. Bupropion is contraindicated in patients with a seizure disorder. To minimize the possibility of seizures, the drug should be given in divided doses and no single dose should exceed 150 mg. Side effects include agitation, insomnia, nausea, tremor, and dry mouth.

Recent clinical experience suggests that psychostimulants may be promising for treating depression with concomitant cognitive impairment in patients with AIDS and ARC. Methylphenidate may be started at doses of 5 mg orally three times a day (0700, 1000, and 1300 hours) and increased by 10–15 mg per day to a maximum dose of 90 mg every 24 hours. If effective, improvement in mood, appetite, energy, and cognition is generally apparent by the third day or at a dose of 45 mg per day. If the depression is nonresponsive to methylphenidate, the medication can be switched to dextroamphetamine (if available) 5–15 mg per day orally in a single morning dose (0800 hours) and then increased by 5–10 mg per day to a maximum of 60 mg every 24 hours in divided doses (0800 and 1200 hours). Contraindications to these stimulants include a history of stimulant abuse, ongoing substance abuse, recent myocardial infarction, and moderate to severe hypertension.

Mania and hypomania may herald the onset of a dementing process. Mania associated with zidovudine administration has been reported. When there is a question regarding the cause, zidovudine should be stopped and the patient observed for any change in manic symptoms. Once treatable organic causes such as central nervous system cryptococcosis have been ruled out, florid organic manic episodes are often successfully treated with antipsychotics and lithium carbonate. Because some patients with AIDS appear to be more vulnerable to the central nervous system toxicity of lithium, it is prudent to aim for an initial serum blood level of 0.5–1.0 mEq/L. After a patient has been stabilized on lithium, zidovudine can be resumed. Carbamazepine may also be effective in treating mania, but its ability to cause leukopenia can cause a problem for patients with low white blood cell counts. Clonazepam (0.5–3 mg per day) is a benzodiazepine with a long half-life which can be substituted for or added to the regimen for treating mania if lithium or neuroleptics are inadequate or produce intolerable side effects. Patients taking clonazepam should be monitored for excessive sedation. In addition to the psychotic features associated with AIDS dementia complex, acute psychoses also can occur. An individual with new onset of psychosis requires immediate psychiatric evaluation and treatment. To treat disabling anxiety that is unresponsive to cognitive-behavioral therapy, short- to intermediate-acting benzodiazepines, such as oxazepam or lorazepam, on a time-limited basis are recommended.

Psychiatric diagnosis is often difficult in patients with AIDS because of the combination or organic mental disorders and strong emotional reactions to lethal illness. These aspects are not mutually exclusive; when they coexist, both need to be addressed in the overall treatment plan. An organic cause of mental status changes should be suspected in all HIV-infected patients before concluding that the symptoms are solely part of a functional syndrome such as an adjustment disorder.

REFERENCES

1. Centers for Disease Control. Classification system for human T lymphotropic virus type III/lymphadenopathy virus type III infections. *MMWR* 1986;35: 334–339.
2. Redfield RR, Wright DC, Tramont EC. The Walter Reed staging classification for HTLV-III/LAV infection. *N Engl J Med* 1986;314:131–132.
3. Kovacs JA, Masur H. *Pneumocystic carinii* pneumonia: Therapy and prophylaxis. *J Infect Dis* 1988;158:254–259.
4. Centers for Disease Control. Guidelines for prophylaxis against *Pneumocystis carinii* pneumonia for persons infected with human immunodeficiency virus. *MMWR* 1989;38(S-5):1–9.
5. Young LS. *Mycobacterium avium* complex infection. *J Infect Dis* 1988;157:863–867.
6. Jacobson MA, Mills J. Serious cytomegalovirus disease in the acquired immunodeficiency syndrome. *Ann Intern Med* 1988;108:585–594.
7. Krown SE. AIDS-assocated Kaposi's sarcoma: Pathogenesis, clinical course, and treatment. *AIDS* 1988;2:71–80.
8. Navia BA, Jordan BD, Price RW. The AIDS dementia complex: I. Clinical features. *Ann Neurol* 1986;19:517–524.
9. Fernandez F, Holmes VF, Levy JK, Ruiz P. Consultation-liaison psychiatry and HIV-related disorders. *Hosp and Comm Psych* 1989;40:146–153.
10. Folstein MF, Folstein SE, McHugh PR. "Mini-mental state"—A practical method for grading the cognitive state of patients for the clinician. *J Psych Res* 1975;12:189–198.

ADDITIONAL READING

Chaisson RE, Slutkin G. Tuberculosis and human immunodeficiency virus infection. *J Infect Dis* 1989;159:96–100.

Dalakas M, Wichman A, Sever J. AIDS and the nervous system. *JAMA* 1989;261:2396–2399.

Glatt AE, Chirgwin K, Landesman SH. Treatment of infections associated with human immunodeficiency virus. *N Engl J Med* 1988;318:1439–1448 .

Hook EW. Syphilis and HIV infection. *J Infect Dis* 1989;160:530–534.

Mills J. *Pneumocystis carinii* and *Toxoplasma gondii* infections in patients with AIDS. *Rev Infect Dis* 1986;8:1001–1011.

Moss AR, Bacchetti P. Natural history of HIV infection. *AIDS* 1989;3:55–61.

Safai B, Lynfield R, Lowenthal DA, Koziner B. Cancers associated with HIV infection. *Anticancer Res* 1987;7:1055–1068.

Tindall B, Barker S, Donovan B, et al. Characterization of the acute clinical illness associated with human immunodeficiency virus infection. *Arch Intern Med* 1988;148:945–949.

Whimbey E, Gold JWM, Polsky B, et al. Bacteremia and fungemia in patients with the acquired immunodeficiency syndrome. *Ann Intern Med* 1986;104:511–514.

Wolcott DL, Fawzy FI, Pasnau RO. Acquired immune deficiency syndrome (AIDS) and consultation-liaison psychiatry. *Gen Hosp Psych* 1985;7:280–292.

Young FE, Norris JA, Levitt JA, Nightingale SL. The FDA's new procedures for the use of investigational drugs in treatment. *JAMA* 1988;259:2267–2270.

Zuger A, Louie E, Holzman RS, et al. Cryptococcal disease in patients with the acquired immunodeficiency syndrome. *Ann Intern Med* 1986;104:234–240.

9

Management of Common Syndromes in Patients with HIV Infection and AIDS

Joseph F. O'Neill
John Mills

From the point of view of a primary care physician, the possibility or fact that a patient is infected with HIV or has AIDS markedly affects the differential diagnosis of a given symptom. Likewise, it changes the workup necessary to evaluate some complaints appropriately, alters the approach to health maintenance, and may mandate new therapeutic approaches to certain routine problems. Management of persons with asymptomatic HIV infection (see Chap. 7) and the approach to many of the complications of HIV infection (see Chap. 8) are discussed elsewhere. This chapter focuses on several common clinical syndromes associated with HIV infection and AIDS and describes their differential diagnosis, evaluation, and initial management. These guidelines are based in part on preliminary recommendations from the World Health Organization.

DIARRHEA

Both acute and chronic diarrhea are relatively common in persons with HIV infection. We define acute diarrhea as more than three liquid stools per day for 2 or more days or a marked or sudden increase in bowel frequency or liquidity in a patient with chronic diarrhea. Chronic diarrhea is defined as more than three to five liquid stools per day for more than 1 month or episodic loose stools. There are limited data regarding the costs and benefits

Table 9-1. Infectious agents and therapy for diarrhea in HIV-infected patients

Organism	Therapy	Comments
Campylobacter jejuni	Erythromycin *or* tetracycline *or* ciprofloxacin	Optimal duration of therapy unknown; 7–21 days
Cryptosporidium	NET	—
CMV	Ganciclovir*	Use restricted to severe or life-threatening disease
Entamoeba histolytica	Metronidazole followed by iodoquinol	Asymptomatic carriers may not merit treatment
Giardia lamblia	Metronidazole *or* quinacrine	No maintenance therapy needed
Isospora belli	Trimethoprim-sulfamethoxazole	Maintenance therapy needed
Microsporidium	NET	—
Mycobacterium avium complex	NET	Multidrug regimens are being studied and appear promising
Mycobacterium tuberculosis	Isoniazid, rifampin, and pyrazinamide	Standard regimen
Salmonella (non-*typhi*)	Trimethoprim-sulfamethoxazole *or* ampicillin *or* ciprofloxacin	7–21 days; relapse is common, and chronic therapy may be needed
Shigella	Trimethoprim-sulfamethoxazole *or* ampicillin *or* ciprofloxacin	7–21 days; relapse is common, and chronic therapy may be needed
Strongyloides stercoralis	Thiabendazole	—

Note: NET = no effective therapy known.
*Not FDA approved for this indication.

of comprehensive gastrointestinal workups in patients with diarrhea. Careful, comprehensive evaluation usually leads to a specific diagnosis, but it is less clear that the majority of identified conditions can be improved by therapy. Some conditions are clearly treatable, however, and an initial evaluation is appropriate for all patients with diarrhea. The most common causes of diarrhea in HIV-infected patients are infectious, including bacterial, viral, and parasitic pathogens (Table 9-1). In one study that involved comprehensive gastrointestinal evaluations, CMV was the leading cause identified.[1] Unfortunately, few clinical features differentiate one cause of enteritis from another, and multiple pathogens may be present simultaneously or sequentially in a patient. However, epidemiologic characteristics of a patient may help to narrow the differential diagnosis. For example, in the developed world, infection with enteric bacteria or protozoa is more prevalent among homosexual men than among heterosexuals. In addition, malignancies, including non-Hodgkin's lymphoma and Kaposi's sarcoma, can cause gastrointestinal symptoms.

Regardless of the cause, the first priority in the management of a patient with diarrhea is supportive care. Evaluation should include staging fluid volume; measuring electrolyte concentrations, especially serum potassium; and replenishing fluid and electrolytes, if appropriate. Hospitalization may be required for fluid and electrolyte repletion if patients are severely dehydrated. Once a patient is stabilized, a comprehensive history and physical examination, including a history of travel, diet, pet exposure, and medications, is warranted. An evaluation of stool for blood, bacteria, ova, and parasites is indicated. Multiple (two to three) stools should be collected for the ova and parasite examinations, preferably on different days. Some laboratories will routinely examine stool for the parasite *Cryptosporidium,* but in other laboratories this test needs to be specifically requested. If the patient is febrile, blood samples for bacterial and mycobacterial cultures should be obtained. If the patient was treated with antibiotics in the past, evaluation of stool for the presence of *Clostridium difficile* or *C. difficile* toxin is appropriate. In the case of chronic diarrhea, an abrupt worsening of symptoms may suggest that periodic repetition of some tests is indicated if the first evaluations are negative. If these initial studies are negative, additional studies may be warranted, depending upon the severity and persistence of the patient's symptoms and underlying condition. Sigmoidoscopy or colonoscopy with biopsy of any inflamed areas or ulcers may be considered in chronic diarrhea, as should visualization, biopsy, or x-ray of the small bowel. These procedures (to look for neoplasms, microsporidia, or CMV) should be used only when noninvasive workup of the patient with chronic diarrhea does not reveal a treatable cause. Diarrhea is, however, an inconsistent symptom of gastrointestinal Kaposi's sarcoma. Formal evaluation for malabsorption, including fecal fat studies, is sometimes useful in order to provide optimal nutritional support.

While awaiting the results of stool examination, a trial of palliative measures such as a clear liquid diet, low-lactose diet, increased bran intake, or decreased fruit intake should be considered. Many persons with AIDS have a marginal nutritional status, and ensuring adequate caloric intake is important. Use of easily digested nutritional supplements or, rarely, parenteral hyperalimentation may be appropriate for selected patients. Opiate constipating agents should not be used if blood or leukocytes are present in the stool and if bacterial or amebic colitis is a likely diagnosis. In general, specific treatment of diarrhea should be directed by the results of the previously described investigations, and empiric therapy should be avoided. However, if blood or leukocytes are present in stool samples, or if a patient has high fever or rigors, antibiotic therapy should be initiated presumptively while awaiting culture results. A drug with activity against *Shigella, Salmonella,* and *Campylobacter,* such as ciprofloxacin (500 mg twice daily) should be selected. If bacterial culture or microscopy identifies a specific organism, therapy should be modified accordingly (Table 9-1). *Salmonella* and *Shigella* infections in this population often recur, even after appropriate initial therapy. If this occurs, a 6- to 12-week course of therapy (e.g., trimethoprim-sulfamethoxazole, one dose twice daily) should be undertaken and chronic suppressive therapy begun. If examination of stool reveals *Giardia lamblia,* therapy with metronidazole (500 mg three times a day for 7 days) or quinacrine should be given. The significance of *Entamoeba histolytica* in stools of asymptomatic persons is unclear because of variability in this organism's pathogenicitiy, but the condition should be treated if found in association with gastrointestinal symptoms. *Isospora belli* oocysts may be found in some patients. This infection often responds well to oral trimethoprim-sulfamethoxazole, but lifelong prophylaxis is usually required to prevent relapse. Cryptosporidial diarrhea is a major management problem. Although there are anecdotal reports of improvement with spiramycin, diclazuril, or bovine transfer factor, there is currently no known effective, specific treatment for this infection in patients with AIDS. If CMV is demonstrated histologically in a patient with invasive colitis, a trial of ganciclovir (10 mg/kg per day for 2 weeks for adults with normal renal function) or foscarnet should be considered (see Chap. 8 for additional details regarding the use of ganciclovir).

RESPIRATORY CONDITIONS

Most patients with AIDS will develop pulmonary symptoms, such as cough, chest pain, or dyspnea. These symptoms are most often due to lower respiratory tract infection, which can be caused by a variety of pathogens, the most common of which are listed in Table 9-2. The clinical presentation and initial evaluation sometimes can suggest the most likely diagnoses. In persons with severe HIV-associated immunodeficiency, as manifested by CD4 lymphocyte counts of less than 200/mm^3, PCP is the most common cause of pneumonia in patients not receiving prophylaxis for PCP[2, 3] (see Chap. 8 for a discussion of the management of PCP). If persons are receiving PCP prophylaxis, PCP can occur but is less likely, and the clinical presentation is often atypical, with unusual radiographic findings (e.g.,

Table 9-2. Causes of and therapy for pulmonary infections in HIV-infected patients

Organism	Therapy	Comments
CMV	Ganciclovir†	Use restricted to severe or life-threatening disease
Endemic fungi *Cryptococcus neoformans* *Histoplasma capsulatum* *Coccidioides immitis*	Amphotericin B	Use of fluconazole and itraconazole is under investigation; ketoconazole used for chronic therapy in selected infections
Legionella sp.	Erythromycin†	Not common
Mycobacterium avium complex	NET	Multidrug regimens are being studied
Mycobacterium tuberculosis	Isoniazid, rifampin, and pyrazinamide	Standard regimen
Pneumocystis carinii	Trimethoprim-sulfamethoxazole *or* pentamidine	See Chap. 8
Pyogenic bacteria*	Standard antimicrobial agent	—
Toxoplasma gondii	Pyrimethamine with sulfadiazine *or* clindamycin	Lifelong suppressive therapy needed

Note: NET = no effective therapy known.
*Especially *Streptococcus pneumoniae* and *Haemophilus influenzae*.
†Not FDA approved for this indication.

apical infiltrates) or extrapulmonary infection. In HIV-infected persons with less immunologic impairment, as manifested by higher CD4 cell counts, PCP is unusual and other causes should be more seriously considered. Tuberculosis can occur as a first opportunistic infection in HIV-infected persons, and radiographic findings are frequently atypical. Pyogenic bacteria, especially encapsulated organisms such as *Streptococcus pneumoniae* and *Haemophilus influenzae,* are common causes of pulmonary disease in any stage of HIV infection.[4] Pneumonia due to coliform bacteria or *Pseudomonas* may occur in terminally ill patients.

In addition to infections, other diseases can occur in the lung (Table 9-3). Kaposi's sarcoma occasionally causes pulmonary disease without cutaneous disease and may present with hemoptysis. The incidence of nonspecific interstitial pneumonitis in persons with AIDS is not entirely clear, but its

Table 9-3. Noninfectious pulmonary processes in AIDS

Organism	Comment
Kaposi's sarcoma	Usually associated with cutaneous disease
Lymphoid interstitial pneumonitis	More common in children than in adults
Lymphoma	—
Nonspecific interstitial pneumonitis	Lung biopsy required for diagnosis
Pleural effusion or empyema	Usually secondary to tuberculosis, bacterial infection, or neoplasm
Pneumothorax	Associated with tuberculosis or PCP

presentation often mimics that of PCP, with a subacute course of cough and dyspnea.

Because presenting complaints in these conditions can be subtle and nonspecific, clinicians should thoroughly investigate any pulmonary complaint in HIV-infected patients. The initial diagnostic approach should include a chest x-ray, arterial blood gas measurements, and sputum examination. If a patient is febrile, blood cultures should be done. These are often sufficient to make a diagnosis and should be reviewed before additional procedures are undertaken. Depending upon the severity of presenting symptoms and signs and the speed with which test results are available, empiric therapy may be appropriate. For example, if chest x-ray reveals an interstitial infiltrate, it is prudent to begin therapy for PCP even if full workup (sputum induction, bronchoalveolar lavage, or bronchoscopy) is incomplete. Likewise, if pyogenic infection is suspected, empiric treatment should be given pending definitive diagnosis. The most common means of diagnosing PCP is by examining sputum induced by inhalation of hypertonic saline or by bronchoalveolar lavage. Pulmonary samples, regardless of the type, should be evaluated for bacteria and mycobacteria, as well as for *P. carinii*. If a patient has pulmonary symptoms with a normal chest x-ray and oxygenation, noninvasive studies such as pulmonary function tests (especially measurement of diffusion capacity) or a gallium scan should be performed to clarify the need for more invasive studies such as bronchoscopy, transbronchoscopic lung biopsy, or percutaneous pleural biopsy.

If the patient is symptomatic with breathlessness or is hypoxemic (arterial pO_2 less than 70 mmHg), supplemental oxygen should be administered. As evaluation proceeds, discussion should begin about the possible causes, course, and outcome of pneumonia in patients with HIV and AIDS. The likelihood that respiratory failure will develop depends upon the cause of the problem. Only a few years ago, the outcome for persons with HIV infection and PCP who required ventilatory support was dismal (approximately 15 percent survival), but more recent data suggest survival rates closer to 40 percent. However, the appropriateness of aggressive support depends upon the patient's underlying condition and wishes; discussion of these issues with patients is almost always indicated. In general, a definitive diagnosis should be established for HIV-infected persons with pneumonia because of the multiple potential causes with differing therapies and the potential toxicities of unnecessary treatments.

Treatment of other pulmonary infections is based upon bacteriologic, cytologic, or histologic evidence (Table 9-2). The presence of acid-fast bacilli in sputum or other pulmonary specimens may indicate infection with *Mycobacterium tuberculosis* or other mycobacteria such as *M. avium* complex. This finding warrants empiric treatment for tuberculosis until speciation of the organism has been completed. A minimum of three drugs is recommended. Infections due to *M. avium* complex are often not treated, although there are some reports suggesting clinical improvement with multidrug regimens. Bacterial infections are treated according to standard approaches. Amphotericin B (0.5–0.7 mg/kg per day IV) or fluconazole (200–400 mg per day) is used for fungal infections. Itraconazole is another promising (investigational) antifungal therapy. Neoplastic lesions are treated with chemotherapy or radiotherapy, if appropriate.

HEADACHE

Although common, the development of headache in an HIV-seropositive individual warrants close scrutiny by the health care provider. The type of headache that demands investigation is one which persists for more than 2 weeks, is severe or rapidly worsening, or is not relieved by a mild analgesic agent. The coincident occurrence of fever is worrisome, but its absence does not eliminate the possibility of an intracranial opportunistic infection. The differential diagnosis includes common causes of headache such as tension, migraine, sinusitis, refractive errors, severe anemia, uncontrolled hypertension, or headache as a side effect of medication (e.g., zidovudine), as well as opportunistic infections and malignancies[5] (Table 9-4) (see also Chap. 8). It is not unusual to have multiple processes, each of which can cause headache, occurring simultaneously in these patients.

In all cases, a careful general and neurologic history should be obtained and an examination performed. If this and routine blood studies (including a complete blood cell count) do not suggest a cause, a brain imaging study (CT or MR) should be done. If any new abnormalities are detected by neurologic examination, a lumbar puncture should be performed expeditiously unless it is clear that the abnormalities are chronic or that focal

Table 9-4. Causes of headache in HIV-infected patients

HIV infection
Viral meningoencephalitis
Lymphoma
Mycobacterium tuberculosis meningitis
Toxoplasma gondii meningoencephalitis
Treponema pallidum
Cryptococcus neoformans meningitis

neurologic abnormalities are present. In the latter instance, brain imaging (CT or MR) to look for a mass lesion should be done first, as the presence of such a lesion is a contraindication to lumbar puncture. If a lumbar puncture is done, cerebrospinal fluid evaluation should include a cell count, microscopy, culture (mycobacterial, bacterial, and fungal), protein and glucose determinations, cryptococcal antigen assay, and VDRL test. In some patients, cerebrospinal fluid virus cultures or cytology may be useful. Blood cultures (bacterial and fungal) should be done in all patients suspected of having meningitis. Management should also include appropriate analgesia and supportive care. Treatment should be based upon the findings of the above studies (see Chap. 8).

LYMPHADENOPATHY

Regional or generalized lymphadenopathy frequently occurs in persons with HIV infection. Persistent generalized lymphadenopathy (defined as two or more separate lymph node groups, with nodes larger than 1 cm in diameter, persisting for more than 1 month, and with no local, contiguous, or systemic infection other than HIV to explain the adenopathy) is a common finding in HIV-infected persons. Although there are multiple causes of lymphadenopathy (Table 9-5) the majority of cases will be due to HIV infection itself. Several of the steps necessary to determine the cause of lymphadenopathy should be routinely done in any HIV-infected individual. These include serologic tests for syphilis and tuberculin skin testing (with controls). If these tests are negative, constitutional symptoms are absent or limited to stable, infrequent night sweats, and there has been no recent enlargement in individual nodes, observation without additional evaluation is appropriate. In contrast, if these conditions are not met, further evaluation is warranted. The next steps generally include a chest x-ray (to look for evidence of granulomatous disease) and lymph node aspiration or biopsy. In experienced

Table 9-5. Causes of lymphadenopathy in HIV-infected patients

Chronic pyoderma
Seborrheic dermatitis
HIV
Kaposi's sarcoma
Lymphoma
Mycobacterium tuberculosis
Cryptococcus neoformans
Histoplasma capsulatum
Toxoplasma gondii
Treponema pallidum

hands, fine-needle aspiration of lymph nodes for culture and cytology can provide almost as much information as can biopsy, although the amount of material required for comprehensive evaluation may require multiple aspirations. Abdominal CT scan may be required for visualization of intraabdominal lymphadenopathy. Treatment is based upon the diagnosis.

DERMATOLOGIC SYMPTOMS

Numerous skin conditions have been described in association with HIV infection.[6] Some of these conditions, including chronic prurigo and urticaria, severe seborrhea, generalized erythroderma, and severe psoriasis, have been attributed to HIV itself, while others are due to superinfection. Varicella-zoster virus, herpes simplex virus, molluscum contagiosum, and human papillomavirus are the most common causes of viral infections of the skin in patients with HIV. In addition, bacterial infections such as furunculosis, impetigo, pyoderma, hidradenitis suppurativa, pyomyositis, syphilis, and disseminated cat scratch disease, as well as fungal infections such as candidosis, dermatophytoses, cryptococcus, histoplasmosis, and sporotrichosis, may involve the skin. Amebiasis cutis and cutaneous leishmaniasis have also been reported in HIV-infected patients. Common noninfectious dermatologic complications include Kaposi's sarcoma and skin eruptions due to drug reactions.

Skin disease in the HIV-infected patient often can be diagnosed by the history and physical examination alone, although there are situations when biopsy or cultures are necessary. If a diagnosis is in question, is significant enough to warrant toxic therapy (e.g., Kaposi's sarcoma), or if the skin does not respond to therapy as expected, skin biopsy is appropriate. In addition to routine stains, a Warthin Starry stain should be done on specimens in which syphilis or cat scratch disease are diagnostic possibilities. Cultures for bacteria may be useful to determine the presence and antimicrobial susceptibility of staphylococci. A serologic test for syphilis is indicated for all patients with rash. When varicella-zoster or herpes simplex virus infection is suspected, a specimen for a fluorescent antibody test and virus culture will support a diagnosis. Specimens for a fluorescent antibody test and culture should be taken from intact vesicles by opening the lesion and obtaining cellular material on a swab that is placed in transport media.

Therapies for dermatologic complaints should be directed at the underlying cause, if identifiable. Because multiple problems may be present simultaneously and necessitate multiple therapies, the simplest regimen possible should be devised. It is unclear if anti-HIV therapy improves the conditions suspected of being causally related to HIV. For pruritis, symptomatic therapy with a nonsedating antihistamine and emollients is appropriate. Seborrheic dermatitis is usually managed by the use of selenium- or tar-containing shampoo and judicious use of topical steroids. Multidermatomal or disseminated varicella-zoster infection should be treated with oral acyclovir (800 mg five times per day) until new lesions have stopped forming and old lesions have scabbed. Treatment of unidermatomal disease, unless it involves the eye, is of uncertain benefit. Intravenous therapy (7.5–10 mg/kg every 8 hours) is warranted for patients with extensive cutaneous dissemination or visceral involvement. Severe herpes simplex virus episodes are treated with oral acyclovir (400 mg three times per day for 7–10 days or until healed). Suppressive therapy with acyclovir (200–400 mg two to three times per day) is indicated in patients with severe disease or frequent recurrences to prevent recurrent herpes simplex virus infections. If the lesions do not heal promptly, acyclovir-resistant virus should be suspected and an infectious disease specialist consulted. Bacterial superinfection of lesions does occur, especially in the perirectal area, and concurrent antibiotic therapy may be necessary. Cryotherapy with liquid nitrogen or opening isolated lesions is the treatment for molluscum contagiosum. Condyloma acuminatum may be treated with liquid nitrogen, topical podophyllin, electrocautery, or surgical excision, depending upon the extent and severity of lesions; however, the recurrence rate is high. Systemic interferon-alpha (2 million units/m^2 per day) may be a beneficial adjunctive therapy. Folliculitis and cellulitis should be treated with a penicillinase-resistant penicillin (e.g., dicloxacillin, 500 mg daily); furuncles or abscesses require incision and drainage and oral or parenteral antibiotics, depending upon their severity. Dermal candidosis is treated with topical nystatin or oral ketoconazole, and dermatophyte infections are treated with topical antifungal agents or oral ketoconazole. Aside from cases of pulmonary involvement, Kaposi's sarcoma is thought to be a cause of death in only a minority of patients, and management varies with the extent of disease and the patient's immunologic condition. If treatment of Kaposi's sarcoma is elected, referral to an oncologist may be warranted to guide in selecting the most appropriate therapy.

VISUAL CHANGES

Visual symptoms in a patient with HIV infection require prompt investigation because of the possibility of sight-threatening CMV retinitis.[7] A careful and complete retinal examination with dilatation of the patient's eyes is essential. If satisfactory examination is not possible or if abnormalities are found, urgent referral to an ophthalmologist is indicated. CMV chorioretinitis typically appears as granular white regions ("exudates") with hemorrhage, frequently in a perivascular distribution. "Cotton wool" spots are also commonly seen in HIV-infected patients but do not produce visual symptoms. If CMV retinal involvement is diagnosed, the patient should receive long-term antiviral therapy with ganciclovir or foscarnet (see Chap 8). Other less common causes of visual changes in persons with HIV include syphilis, toxoplasmosis, herpes simplex virus, and varicella-zoster infection (Table 9–6). Eyelid closure secondary to periorbital edema from Kaposi's sarcoma also may compromise vision. In addition to ophthalmologic evaluation, persons with visual complaints should undergo a neurologic examination. If a visual field defect is documented, an MR or CT scan of the brain is indicated. Depending upon the diagnostic possibilities, appropriate evaluations may include serologic tests for toxoplasma and syphilis, buffy coat and urine cultures for CMV, or other virus cultures.

FEVER

The acute and chronic phases of HIV infection, opportunistic complications, and some therapies can cause fever in the HIV-infected patient. Exhaustive

Table 9-6. Causes of visual changes in HIV-infected patients

CMV
Varicella-zoster virus
Herpes simplex virus
Kaposi's sarcoma
Toxoplasma gondii (central nervous system or retina)
Treponema pallidum

workup of every temperature elevation in every patient would generate needless expense. Conversely, fever should not be ignored, as it can be a marker of a significant change in health status. The overriding considerations in the assessment of a patient with HIV who has a fever should be the likelihood of finding a cause that can be treated and of providing palliation. Round-the-clock antipyretics may help blunt extreme temperature fluctuations and minimize discomfort.

It is helpful to think of fever in this population as being either acute or chronic. In most cases, a marked change in the pattern of chronic fever can be approached in the same way as an new, acute fever. The first step in evaluating an acute fever is a careful review of systems, review of current medications, and a physical examination. Particular attention should be paid to respiratory and neurologic systems for signs or symptoms suggestive of pneumonia or central nervous system infection. *P. carinii* infection can present with fever alone; therefore, a chest x-ray is indicated as part of the evaluation of fever. In patients with extrapulmonary pneumocystosis, fever may be the only finding. In the absence of localizing symptoms or signs, CBC with white blood cell differential count, liver function tests, and blood cultures (bacterial, fungal, and mycobacterial) should be done. Additional steps would be directed by the results of the physical examination and the review of systems. If these studies are nonrevealing and fever persists, consideration should be given to urinalysis, urine culture, buffy coat culture for CMV, cerebrospinal fluid evalution, or abdominal CT scan. Maintaining appropriate fluid intake and, if possible, adequate nutritional intake is important. A patient with chronic fever should be encouraged to maintain a temperature record to detect alterations in pattern. Symptomatic measures including antipyretics can be used, but careful attention should be paid to new signs or symptoms.

REFERENCES

1. Smith PD, Land C, Gioll VJ. Intestinal infection in patients with AIDS: Etiology and response to therapy. *Ann Intern Med* 1988;108:328–333.
2. Hopewell PC. *Pneumocystis carinii* pneumonia: Diagnosis. *J Infect Dis* 1988;157:1115–1119.
3. Kovacs JA, Masur H. *Pneumocystis carinii* pneumonia: Therapy and prophylaxis. *J Infect Dis* 1988;158:254–259.
4. Schrager LK. Bacterial infections in AIDS patients. *AIDS* 1988;2(suppl 1):S183–189.
5. McArthur J. Neurologic manifestations of AIDS. *Medicine* (Baltimore) 1987;66:407–436.
6. Sindrup JH, Lisby G, Weismann K, et al. Skin manifestations in AIDS, HIV infection, and AIDS-related complex. *Int J Derm* 1987;26:267–272.

7. Jacobson MA, Mills J. Serious cytomegalovirus disease in the acquired immunodeficiency syndrome. *Ann Intern Med* 1988;108:585–594.

ADDITIONAL READING

Gazzard B. HIV Disease and the gastroenterologist. *Gut* 1988;29:1497–1505.

Holander H. Practical management of common AIDS-related medical problems. *West J Med* 1987;146:237–240.

Krown SE. AIDS-associated Kaposi's sarcoma: Pathogenesis, clinical course, and treatment. *AIDS* 1988;2:71–80.

Leoung GS, Mills J. *Opportunistic infections in patients with the acquired immunodeficiency syndrome*. New York: Marcel Dekker, Inc., 1989.

Pape JW. Treatment of gastrointestinal infections. *AIDS* 1988;2(suppl 1):S161–167.

Pitchenik AE. The treatment and prevention of mycobacterial disease in patients with HIV infection. *AIDS* 1988;2(suppl):S177–182.

Sande M, Volberding P. *The medical management of AIDS*. Philadelphia: W. B. Saunders, 1988.

10

HIV Infection in Pregnancy and Infancy

Heather Watts
Sandra Burchett

PREGNANCY

Women now comprise 9 percent of the cases of AIDS reported in the United States, and 80 percent of women with AIDS are of reproductive age (15–44 years). The demographics of HIV infection would be expected to be similar to those of AIDS; thus there is a large reservoir of asymptomatic, seropositive women of childbearing age who may transmit the infection to their infants and who themselves may later become ill. Surveys of pregnant women and newborn infants have shown HIV seroprevalences ranging from 0.9 to 12.5 per 1000, with rates being highest among urban minority women.[1, 2] Among pregnant drug users studied in Baltimore, the prevalence of HIV antibody positivity was 30 percent. Eighty percent of pediatric AIDS cases are secondary to perinatal transmission of the virus. IV drug use by women or their partners remains the most common risk factor for maternal and infant infection; 53 percent of the 1087 cases of perinatally acquired AIDS cases reported in the United States through January 1989 occurred in children born to women who used IV drugs, and 20 percent were children born to partners of men who used IV drugs.

As the AIDS epidemic increases, all health care providers must become familiar with procedures for screening, counseling, and caring for patients potentially infected with HIV. HIV infection in pregnant women presents unique issues, which can be considered in the context of the antepartum, intrapartum, and postpartum periods.

Antepartum issues

An important question in the antepartum period is how and when to screen for HIV infection. Preliminary studies have shown that up to one-half of

HIV-seropositive pregnant women either had no identifiable risk factors for HIV infection or were unaware of their high-risk status.[1] Thus, screening programs based on detecting and screening only women known to be at high risk (Table 10-1) may miss a large number of infected women. Currently, it is recommended that all pregnant women be offered HIV screening as part of prenatal care. This screening must be accompanied by specific pre- and posttest counseling (see Chap. 6) to ensure education about HIV infection. Women should never be screened without their knowledge and consent. Seronegative pregnant women who engage in high-risk behaviors should be educated about reducing their risk; if they continue to engage in such behaviors, they should be rescreened during their third trimester.

Seropositive women require additional evaluation and counseling. A woman's potential responses to a positive test result must be assessed during pretest counseling so that appropriate support mechanisms can be available when she receives her test result. In addition to the usual posttest counseling appropriate for any HIV-seropositive person, the issues specific to HIV infection in pregnancy must be discussed (Table 10-2). The 20–50 percent risk of perinatal transmission must be clearly explained.[3] Although early studies estimated a 50–60 percent risk of transmission of HIV from mother to infant, the women studied were in advanced stages of HIV infection or had previously given birth to a child who developed AIDS. Thus, these women were probably selected as being those most likely to transmit the infection to their offspring. Subsequent studies have shown transmission rates of 20–40 percent for asymptomatic, HIV-positive women. Possible exceptions to the lower rate are women who develop acute HIV infection during pregnancy; such women are more likely to have high-level viremia and transmission rates may be higher, although few women in this circumstance have been evaluated. If a seropositive woman is at less than 24 weeks of gestation, she should be informed of the option of terminating the pregnancy to prevent perinatal transmission. We believe that counseling should be informative and nondirective, and that women should be supported regardless of their choice. Reports to date have shown that the majority of HIV-seropositive women elect to continue their pregnancy.[4]

Seropositive women should be educated regarding transmission of HIV; instructed in safer sexual practices, including the use of condoms during pregnancy; and instructed not to share needles. They should be informed of the need for partner notification and assisted in this task. Although the limited data available have not shown an adverse effect of HIV infection on the outcome of pregnancy in asymptomatic women, women who have advanced HIV infection or AIDS may have an increased risk of preterm birth and other adverse outcomes.[5, 6] It is unclear whether pregnancy hastens the progression of HIV-related disease, and there are still no data to support terminating pregnancy for a woman's health. Additionally, no

Table 10-1. Behaviors of women that increase their risk for HIV infection

IV drug use
Sexual partner of an IV drug user
Sexual partner of a bisexual man
Sex with multiple partners
Sex with men with STDs
Blood transfusion recipient during 1978–1985

controlled studies have been conducted to determine whether antiviral therapy, such as zidovudine, may alter the vertical transmission rate. Small numbers of pregnant women have been treated with zidovudine to date. Physicians administering this medication must weigh the potential benefits against the potential adverse effects of zidovudine on a growing fetus. Animal studies do not suggest any teratogenic effect of zidovudine, but studies that would expose many uninfected human fetuses to a potentially toxic drug must be undertaken with great caution. However, if a pregnant woman develops serious HIV-related disease that would indicate a need for antiviral therapy such as zidovudine, the therapy should not be withheld. The optimal dose of zidovudine during pregnancy is unknown (see Chap. 11).

Pregnant women who are HIV seropositive should be screened for other sexually transmitted diseases, including hepatitis B, syphilis, gonorrhea, and *Chlamydia trachomatis* infections (Table 10-3). They need a tuberculin skin test with accompanying anergy panel. Baseline serologic testing for antibody to CMV and *Toxoplasma gondii* is helpful if symptomatic infections with either microorganism develop; then it can be determined whether the infection is primary or recurrent, as the risk to the fetus is

Table 10-2. Issues to be addressed in counseling HIV-seropositive pregnant women

Risk of perinatal transmission (20–50 percent)
Options of continuing or terminating pregnancy
Transmission modes (sex, sharing needles)
Transmission prevention (safer sex practices, condom use, no IV drug use; if drugs are used, clean needles should be employed)
Partner notification

Table 10-3. Evaluating HIV-infected pregnant women

Screen for STDS
Hepatitis B
Syphilis
Neisseria gonorrhoeae infection
Chlamydia trachomatis infection
Tuberculin skin test (with controls)
CMV antibody test
Toxoplasma gondii antibody test
CBC count with the white blood cell differential count
T-lymphocyte subsets (CD4, percent and number)

Note: In addition to routine management.

different for each. Baseline complete blood cell counts and T-lymphocyte testing should also be performed. Women whose CD4 lymphocyte count is greater than 400/mm^3 usually remain asymptomatic but must be followed closely for opportunistic infections or malignancy, as the physiologic changes of pregnancy may mask symptoms or delay the diagnosis of HIV-related disease. Obstetric health care providers who are not familiar with caring for HIV-infected patients should refer pregnant women who are symptomatic, who have CD4 lymphocyte counts less than 400/mm^3, or who would like additional information regarding their condition to a specialist for consultation. For example, women whose CD4 lymphocyte counts are less than 200/mm^3 or who have had previous PCP are at increased risk for PCP, although no suitable prophylactic agents are currently available for use during pregnancy. To ensure appropriate follow-up after delivery, women should be referred to an ongoing primary care provider during pregnancy.

Intrapartum issues

Intrapartum care is the same for seropositive and seronegative pregnant women. Universal body substance isolation procedures should be maintained during delivery to prevent transmission of blood-borne infections (Table 10-4; see also Chap. 14). These precautions include wearing waterproof gowns, masks, gloves, and goggles and handling the baby with gloves until he or she has been bathed. Parenteral therapy for the infant (such as vitamin K) or heelstick hematocrit determinations should be delayed until after stabilization and bathing to avoid inoculation of HIV through the neonate's skin. All needles and sharp instruments must be used carefully;

Table 10-4. Infection control measures during delivery

Latex gloves (until infant is bathed)
Waterproof gowns
Goggles
Masks
Delay injections or blood drawing until infant is bathed

needles should never be recapped and must be disposed of promptly. The mode of delivery is determined by the usual obstetric indications. HIV infection is not an indication for cesarean section, as there is no evidence at present that abdominal delivery either decreases or increases the risk of perinatal HIV transmission. Procedures such as fetal scalp electrode placement and fetal blood sampling, which potentially increase the exposure of fetal blood to maternal secretions, may increase the risk of HIV or other viral transmission and should be avoided when possible.

Postpartum issues

Postpartum care of the HIV-seropositive pregnant woman is similar to that for seronegative women, except that breast feeding should be discouraged if safe alternatives are available. Cases of HIV transmission apparently related to breast feeding have been reported,[7] and in the United States breast feeding in this circumstance is not recommended. In developing nations, where the risks to the infant of diarrhea and other infections are higher, breast feeding is recommended regardless of HIV status. Isolation of HIV-seropositive women is not indicated, although gloves should be worn when handling materials containing secretions. Isolation of the infant in the nursery is not necessary, as HIV-infected neonates do not present a risk to other babies. However, exposure of potentially HIV-infected neonates to babies shedding CMV or other viral pathogens should be avoided. Obviously, the usual handwashing practices in the nursery are important. Postpartum women should be counseled regarding contraceptive alternatives and provided with effective methods for contraception before hospital discharge. Methods that prevent HIV transmission should be encouraged. Follow-up for the seropositive mother should be arranged before discharge from the maternity unit to ensure appropriate management of HIV infection (see Chaps. 7 and 8). Ideally, seropositive women should be referred to a pediatric infectious disease specialist during pregnancy for counseling and follow-up of the infant after delivery.

INFANCY

Epidemiology

Pediatric AIDS cases in the United States reported to the CDC totaled 1355 as of January 1989; of these, 5 percent were infected after treatment for hemophilia and 13 percent were infected by contaminated blood products (Table 10-5). The majority acquired AIDS perinatally, and this group continues to increase in number nationwide. By the end of 1991, an estimated 10,000–20,000 children will have been diagnosed with AIDS. At present, essentially all new cases in children are due to perinatal infection, and the majority are diagnosed in the first year of life. Of the infants with AIDS in the United States, 75 percent are members of a minority group. While children still represent a small proportion of the total number of persons with AIDS, the increase in newly infected children born to HIV-infected mothers reflects the seropositivity rate in drug-using heterosexuals in a given area. Consequently, certain areas, such as New York, New Jersey, and Florida, have a disproportionate share of pediatric AIDS cases.

Diagnosis

Babies born to seropositive mothers will be positive for HIV by traditional antibody testing techniques (ELISA and Western blot) for as long as 15 months after birth because of passive transfer of maternal antibody. Therefore, specialized testing is necessary to identify the 20–40 percent of infants who are infected. Laboratory identification of HIV-infected infants less than 15 months of age requires detection of the virus, not just of antibodies to HIV (Table 10-6). Currently, the majority of virus detection tests are available only on a research basis, and include HIV culture, viral antigen (p24) detection, and detection of HIV by polymerase chain reaction (PCR). By definition, if the infant still is positive by ELISA and Western blot at 15 months of age, he or she is considered infected. However, up to 15 percent

Table 10-5. Risk factors for pediatric AIDS in cases reported to the CDC as of January 1989

Risk factor	No. (%)
Perinatal transmission	1057 (78)
Blood transfusion	176 (13)
Factor concentrate for hemophilia	68 (5)
Other or unknown	54 (4)
Total	1355

Table 10-6. Procedures for laboratory diagnosis of pediatric HIV infection

Serologic	
	Persistently positive ELISA after 15 months of age*
	Appearance of new HIV-specific bands by Western blot
Virologic	
	Positive culture of infant's blood cells
	Positive HIV (p24) antigen in infant's plasma or serum
	Positive HIV PCR from infant's cells

Note: All tests must be performed in a quality controlled, certified laboratory.

*Fifteen percent or less of children will still be positive by ELISA at 15 months but will probably not be infected.

of apparently uninfected children are still antibody positive at 15 months. Development of new HIV bands on sequential Western blots also indicates HIV infection. Antibody-positive infants with AIDS-defining illnesses also meet the CDC's pediatric AIDS case definition even if they are less than 15 months of age (Table 10-7). Seropositive infants should be examined and tested at 2- to 3-month intervals during the first 15 months of life. Repeatedly normal laboratory evaluations in infants who show no signs or symptoms of HIV infection suggest that they are most likely not infected. Preliminary data from the United States suggest that infected neonates may have elevated titers of IgG and IgM, and lower CD4 cell counts than do noninfected infants, but their values still overlap with the normal range. Current data suggest that asymptomatic children born to HIV-infected mothers whose antibody tests become negative have approximately a 1–5 percent chance of being infected. These infected children may develop clinical evidence of HIV infection in future years.

Classification

Pediatric HIV infection is classified by the CDC for surveillance purposes differently from adult disease (Table 10-7).[8] P-O classification includes those infants who are seropositive due to passive transplacental transfer of maternal antibody but whose HIV infection status is not yet clear. An infected child who is asymptomatic but who may have mild abnormalities in laboratory data is classified as P-1. Infants and children with symptomatic infection or AIDS-defining illnesses are classified as P-2. Categories P-1 and P-2 have multiple subcategories.

Table 10-7. Summary of the classification of HIV infection in children less than 13 years of age

Class P-O. Indeterminate infection

Class P-1. Asymptomatic infection
- Subclass A. Nonspecific findings
- Subclass B. Abnormal immune function
- Subclass C. Immune function not tested

Class P-2. Symptomatic infection
- Subclass A. Nonspecific findings
- Subclass B. Progressive neurologic disease
- Subclass C. Lymphoid interstitial pneumonitis
- Subclass D. Secondary infectious diseases
  - Category D-1. Specified secondary infectious diseases listed in the CDC's surveillance definition for AIDS*
  - Category D-2. Recurrent serious bacterial infections
  - Category D-3. Other specified secondary infectious disease
- Subclass E. Secondary cancers
  - Category E-1. Specified secondary cancers listed in the CDC's surveillance definition for AIDS*
  - Category E-2. Other cancers possibly secondary to HIV infection
- Subclass F. Other diseases possibly due to HIV infection

*See Chap. 8.

Source: Centers for Disease Control. Classification system for human immunodeficiency virus (HIV) infection in children under 13 years of age. *MMWR* 1987;36:225–236.

Clinical manifestations and management

The differential diagnosis of children with AIDS includes congenital immunodeficiencies and several congenital infections (CMV, rubella, syphilis, and toxoplasmosis), as well as HIV infection. Clinical care of P-O infants is the same as that of healthy HIV-seronegative infants except for immunization recommendations (Table 10-8)[9]. If a baby is known to be HIV infected, medical and social care intensify. Mild illnesses common in infants can be much more severe in HIV-infected children. These children often present with severe bacterial or opportunistic infections. Additionally, recommendations to prevent potentially life-threatening infections such as CMV differ for the HIV-infected child. Therefore, it is prudent to establish the diagnoses in infected infants as soon as possible. The infant who presents with symptoms and signs suggestive of AIDS should be tested immediately after counseling and consent by the infant's parent(s) or guardian(s), because empiric therapy for the suspected secondary infections in the HIV-infected child differs from that for other children with similar symptoms. For example, empiric therapy for PCP might be used more readily in a child

Table 10-8. CDC Immunization Practices Advisory Committee recommendations for routine immunization of HIV-infected children

	Vaccine						
HIV status	**DPT**	**OPV**	**IPV**	**MMR**	**HbCV**	**Pneumo-coccal**	**Influenza**
Asymptomatic (known)	+	−	+	+	+	−*	−*
Symptomatic	+	−	+	+*	+	+	+

Note: DTP = diphtheria and tetanus toxoids and pertussis vaccine; OPV = oral, attenuated poliovirus vaccine (contains poliovirus types 1, 2, and 3); IPV = inactivated poliovirus vaccine (contains poliovirus types 1, 2, and 3); MMR = live measles, mumps, and rubella viruses (combined vaccine); HbCV = *Hemophilus influenzae* type b conjugate vaccine. + = recommended, − = not recommended.

*Should be considered.

Source: Immunization practices advisory committee. General recommendations on immunization. *MMWR* 1989;38:221–222.

with pneumonia. It is also important to identify the healthy seropositive infant who is at risk of HIV infection but in whom the infection cannot yet be conclusively determined (P-O). Frequently, questions of home placement or adoption arise for these children when their mothers or families are not able to provide care, and testing may facilitate appropriate placement in a nurturing environment. At present there is an urgent need for receiving or foster homes where the care providers are knowledgeable about AIDS. The only reported case of infection of a care provider (including day care workers) for an infected infant is one mother who repeatedly handled bloody secretions carelessly. Handwashing before and after contact with the infant and the use of gloves if the child has diarrhea or bloody secretions should eliminate even the low theoretical risk of transmission to the care provider and decrease the potential of transmitting infections to the infant.

The incubation period for pediatric AIDS is usually much shorter than that for adults. Although a mean of 6 years from infection to diagnosis is found with transfusion-associated cases, this period is usually significantly less (mean, 3 years) in perinatally acquired cases. However, there may be two risk populations for the acquisition of AIDS in perinatally infected children. Many infants will develop AIDS during the first year of life, although rarely in the first 2 months. As many as one-half of these children, if untreated, will die within 8 months after diagnosis, especially if PCP has occurred. The second population seems to develop AIDS at a mean of 6 years; one-half of these children will live longer than 2 years from diagnosis

(Fig. 10-1). Whether the prognosis of these children will change with wider availability of antiviral therapy is unknown.

Infants and children may present with opportunistic infections as the first manifestation of AIDS in a manner similar to that seen in adults. The predominant opportunistic infections are acute PCP, disseminated CMV, or candidal esophagitis (Table 10-9). Malignancies are rare. Common chronic manifestations include persistent oral thrush, failure to thrive, and neurodevelopmental delay or loss of previously acquired developmental milestones. Lymphoid interstitial pneumonitis, uncommon in adults, is frequent in children with AIDS and causes chronic hypoxemic lung disease with a subacute clinical presentation. Treatment for lymphoid interstitial pneumonitis includes oxygen and, in selected cases, corticosteroids. Severe bacterial infections, such as meningitis, sepsis, or pneumonia, are more common in pediatric than in adult cases. Differentiation among the multiple pulmonary presentations is via bronchial alveolar lavage or open lung biopsy.

Treatment of HIV and its complications

Table 10-10 describes the treatment regimens for several common pediatric conditions associated with HIV infection. Antibacterial and antifungal therapies do not differ substantially from those for other pediatric populations. Antiretroviral therapy was recently approved for children less than 13 years of age. Treatment trials are being conducted at centers throughout the

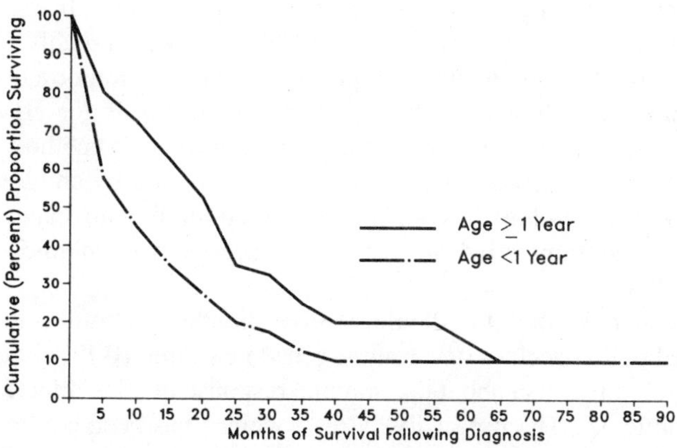

Figure 10-1. Survival time after diagnosis of AIDS in children less than 13 years of age in whom AIDS was diagnosed as of December 31, 1981, and reported to the CDC. (Reprinted by permission from Rogers MF, Thomas PA, Starcher ET, et al. Acquired immunodeficiency syndrome in children: Report of the Centers for Disease Control National Surveillance, 1982 to 1985. *Pediatrics* 1987;79:1008–1014.)

Table 10-9. Relative frequencies of opportunistic diseases and malignancies reported for children with AIDS

Disease or malignancy	Percent occurrence
PCP	53
Lymphoid interstitial pneumonitis	51
Disseminated CMV	19
Candidal esophagitis	19
Disseminated *Mycobacterium avium*	7
Cryptosporidiosis	5
Chronic herpes simplex virus	5
Kaposi's sarcoma	4
Cryptococcosis	1
Toxoplasmosis	1
Progressive multifocal leukoencephalopathy	<1

Source: Adapted from Rogers MF, Thomas PA, Starcher ET, et al. Acquired immunodeficiency syndrome in children: Report of the Centers for Disease Control National Surveillance, 1982 to 1985. *Pediatrics* 1987;79:1008–1014.

United States for children and neonates. Through these trials, zidovudine is available for children with AIDS or symptomatic HIV infection. The dose for children more than 3 months of age is 180 mg/m^2 every 6 hours, whereas the pharmacokinetics and optimal dose for neonates are still under investigation. Preliminary data suggest that zidovudine in children may reduce HIV-associated neurologic manifestations and neurodevelopmental delay.[10] Although controversial, some studies suggest that monthly gamma globulin infusions may decrease the number of severe bacterial infections and, consequently, prolong the life span of infected children. In one ongoing study of zidovudine, children are randomized between monthly IV gamma globulin and placebo in an attempt to answer this important question. Studies have not shown the best prophylaxis for PCP for HIV-infected children. Preliminary data suggest that trimethoprim-sulfamethoxazole, one common form of prophylaxis, is more easily tolerated by children than by adults. IV pentamidine has been used in children who cannot tolerate trimethoprim-sulfamethoxazole. The use of aerosol pentamidine in children is under study.

Infants at risk for HIV should receive diphtheria/pertussis/tetanus and inactivated polio vaccines on a routine schedule (Table 10-8), although there are relatively little data about the immune response of HIV-infected children to these antigens. The use of live virus vaccines has been controversial. A relatively large prospective study of African children with and without HIV infection who received measles vaccine showed that although children infected with HIV were more likely to die from measles than were HIV-negative children, none responded adversely to immunization. Fatal cases of

Table 10-10. Pediatric dosages for AIDS-related therapies

Therapy	Dose	Route of administration
Anti-HIV treatment		
Zidovudine	180 mg/m^2 every 6 hours	PO
PCP treatment		
Trimethoprim-sulfamethoxazole	5 mg trimethoprim/kg every 6 hours for 14 days	IV
or		
Pentamidine isothionate	4mg/kg every day for 14 days	IV
PCP prophylaxis		
Trimethoprim-sulfamethoxazole	75 mg trimethoprim/m^2 every 12 hours	PO
	or	
or	150 mg trimethoprim/m^2 every day	
Pentamidine isothionate	4 mg/kg every 2–4 weeks	IV
	or	
	4 mg/kg every 4 weeks	Aerosol
Antibacterial prophylaxis		
Gamma globulin	400mg/kg every 4 weeks	IV

measles have also occurred in children with and without HIV infection in the United States. Retrospective studies in New York City have documented no adverse events in HIV-infected children who received measles/mumps/rubella or oral polio vaccines. Although HIV-infected children with immunologic dysfunction may not become immune after immunization, the present recommendation is that all infected children receive measles/mumps/rubella vaccine, with the possible exception of those with severe immunologic dysfunction. HIV-infected children should receive *Hemophilus influenzae* type b conjugate vaccine. Pneumococcal and influenza virus vaccines are recommended for symptomatic HIV-infected children and are optional for infected asymptomatic children.

CONCLUSION

As the proportion of newly diagnosed HIV-infected individuals continues to increase in heterosexual women of childbearing age, strategies to prevent vertical transmission of HIV are critical. Effective programs to curtail heterosexual or IV drug–related transmission are vital to help prevent pediatric HIV infections. A comprehensive care system is necessary for HIV-seropositive women and their infants. Early identification of HIV-infected babies is crucial to efficiently diagnose and treat common, opportunistic, or severe bacterial infections and to maximize the benefits of antiviral treatment. Babies and children cannot speak for themselves, but they are subject to every facet of the social, moral, and medical dilemmas of HIV infection. We must remain advocates for the rights of mothers and children to receive medical care and to live a healthy life in a nurturing, nonjudgmental environment.

REFERENCES

1. Landesman S, Minkoff H, Holman S, McCalla S, Sijin O. Serosurvey of human immunodeficiency virus infection in parturients: Implications for HIV testing programs of pregnant women. *JAMA* 1987;258:2701–2703.
2. Hoff R, Berardi VP, Weibein BJ, et al. Seroprevalence of HIV among childbearing women: Estimation by testing samples of blood from newborns. *N Engl J Med* 1988;318:525.
3. Mok JQ, Rossi A, DeAdes A, et al. Infants born to mothers seropositive for human immunodeficiency virus: Preliminary findings from a multicenter European study. *Lancet* 1987;1:1164.
4. Selwyn PA, Schoenbaum EE, Davenny K, et al. Prospective study of HIV infection and pregnancy outcomes in intravenous drug users. *JAMA* 1989;261:1289–1294.
5. Minkoff H, Nanda D, Menez R, Fikring S. Pregnancies resulting in infants with AIDS or AIDS-related complex. *Obstet Gynecol* 1987;69:285.
6. Koonin LM, Ellerbrock TV, Atrash HK, et al. Pregnancy-associated deaths due to AIDS in the United States. *JAMA* 1989;261:1306–1309.
7. Ziegler JB, Cooper DA, Johnson RO, Gold J. Postnatal transmission of AIDS-associated retrovirus from mother to infant. *Lancet* 1985;1:896.
8. Centers for Disease Control. Classification system for human immunodeficiency virus (HIV) infection in children under 13 years of age. *MMWR* 1987;36:225–236.
9. Immunization practices advisory committee. General recommendations on immunization. *MMWR* 1989;38:221–222.
10. Pizzo PA, Eddy J, Falloon J, et al. Effect of continous intravenous infusion of zidovudine (AZT) in children with symptomatic HIV infection. *N Engl J Med* 1988;319:889–896.

ADDITIONAL READING

Auger I, Thomas P, DeGruttola V, et al. Incubation periods for paediatric AIDS patients. *Nature* 1988;336:575–577.

Curran JW, Jaffe HW, Hardy AM, et al. Epidemiology of HIV infection and AIDS in the United States. *Science* 1988;239:610–616.

Falloon J, Eddy J, Wiener L, Pizzo P. Human immunodeficiency virus infection in children. *J Pediatr* 1989;114:1–30.

Minkoff HL. Care of pregnant women infected with HIV. *JAMA* 1987;258:2714–2717.

Pahwa S. Human immunodeficiency virus infection in children: Nature of immunodeficiency, clinical spectrum, and management. *Pediatr Infect Dis J* 1988;7:S61–S71.

11

Antiretroviral Chemotherapy for Treatment of HIV Infection

Teresa A. Tartaglione
Lawrence Corey

The wide distribution of HIV-infected cells in the body combined with the ability of the virus to infect lymphocytes and neuronal cells both latently and productively present enormous challenges for any chemotherapeutic agent. Currently, one effective antiviral drug, zidovudine, is licensed for the treatment of HIV infection. Several other chemotherapeutic agents are currently under clinical investigation and appear promising. Because of the complex replicative cycle of HIV, it is likely that multiple treatment strategies to inhibit HIV activity will be needed to prolong life and decrease the morbidity of this currently inevitably fatal disease. This review focuses on current strategies to treat HIV infection and provides guidelines for the primary physician for use of antiretroviral agents.

TARGETS FOR ANTI-HIV ACTIVITY

The replicative ("life") cycle of HIV follows a set pattern of viral attachment, entry into the host cell, uncoating, replication, and assembly and release from the cell. Each step represents a potential target for antiviral attack (Table 11-1, Fig. 11-1).

Inhibiting attachment or entry of HIV into a cell has theoretical appeal because it would prevent development of both latent and productive infection. Attachment of newly infected cells can be prevented by polyclonal or

Table 11-1. Possible targets for therapeutic intervention in stages of HIV replication

Stage	Possible intervention
Binding to target cell	Antibodies to virus or cellular receptor, recombinant soluble CD4
Entry into target cell and uncoating of RNA	Drugs that block fusion or interfere with retroviral uncoating (soluble CD4, polyionic sulfates)
Transcription of RNA to DNA by reverse transcriptase	Reverse transcriptase inhibitors (zidovudine, ddI, ddC, foscarnet, Azdu)
Degradation of RNA by RNase activity (encoded by viral *pol* gene)	RNase-H inhibitors
Integration of DNA into host genome	Agents that inhibit polymerase-mediated integration (future prospects)
Transcription of DNA to RNA	Specific inhibitors of retroviral transcription have not been developed. However, RNAs that inhibit RNA transcription have been developed. (Anti-HIV-1–specific ribozymes are under development)
Translation of RNA	Inhibitors of genes that enhance retroviral translation, such as *tat, rev,* or *nef*
Viral component production and assembly	Inhibition of viral protease. Inhibitors or modifiers of glycosylation of viral proteins
Viral budding	Interferons

Note: ddI = dideoxyinosine; ddC = dideoxycytidine.

monoclonal antibodies directed against the cell receptors (CD4 molecules) to which the virus attaches, as well as by agents that would block the binding of the viral glycoprotein to the CD4 receptor. One of the enigmas of the pathogenesis of HIV infection is the relatively low titer of neutralizing antibodies seen in humans, even in early stages of disease. Whether this is related to antigenic changes in the virus or to other mechanisms is unclear. Chronic passive immunotherapy with high-titered globulins containing antibodies to the virus produces a transient decrease in the amount of HIV circulating in plasma. However, no trials of chronic therapy with

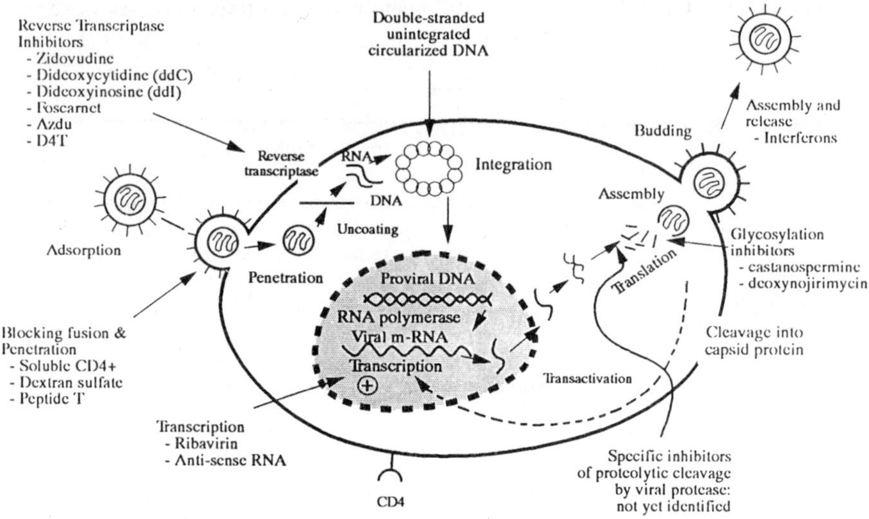

Figure 11-1. The replication cycle of HIV and possible sites of drug action.

such a preparation exist, and whether this approach would be effective clinically is unknown. Large-scale production of human antibodies with high neutralizing capability to a wide variety of HIV strains is not currently available.

Greater attention has been paid to compounds that block the cell receptor for HIV, such as soluble CD4, or alter the attachment process of the viral envelope glycoprotein to the CD4 receptor. Currently under clinical investigation, peptide T is a 10-amino-acid peptide that binds to a region on the CD4 molecule and thereby appears to prevent HIV from entering cells. The polyanionic sulfates, such as dextran sulfate, also inhibit fusion of the HIV virus with cells. Dextran sulfate has been shown in vitro to inhibit HIV and to prevent binding of HIV to T lymphocytes. However, recent pharmacokinetic studies have shown that, as currently manufactured, dextran is not absorbed orally and at high doses (greater than 2 g per day) can cause hepatic toxicity. Studies using dextran sulfate administered IV are underway, and other congeners are under development. Soluble CD4 has been shown to bind strongly with the HIV-1 gp120 and to prevent syncytium formation in cell cultures. As this binding is associated with a conserved region of all HIV-1 and HIV-2 isolates, this therapy offers the potential of inhibiting all clinical isolates of HIV-1. Studies in primates indicate that soluble CD4 may decrease viral replication in animals infected with the simian immunodeficiency virus (SIV). Early phase I trials of soluble recombinant CD4 in humans have shown little toxicity, albeit the half-life of the drug is short. Hooking of CD4 to an immunoglobulin-like molecule such as IgG1 has recently been reported. Thus hybrid molecule (called an *immunoadhesin*) has a very long half-life and offers the potential for achieving high levels of CD4 in plasma for extended periods of time.

After attachment and entry, the next step that could be inhibited in theory is the intracellular uncoating of the virus. No compounds that inhibit this viral process have yet entered clinical trials. However, several compounds have been developed that inhibit the next steps, which involve viral RNA and DNA replication. Reverse transcriptase is a viral enzyme that is essential to HIV replication but has no essential mammalian cell function. Inhibitors of reverse transcriptase, therefore, should act selectively on retroviruses and exhibit an in vivo antiviral effect. Zidovudine appears to be the prototype of compounds with this mechanism of action. While anti-reverse transcriptase inhibitors are effective chemotherapeutic agents, one must remember that reverse transcriptase is not necessary in all parts of the viral cycle. Thus, chronically or persistently infected cells such as monocytes or macrophages will produce infectious virus and not be affected by an inhibitor of reverse transcriptase.

Other potential targets for inhibiting HIV replication include viral integration into host-cell DNA; posttranscriptional processing of viral mRNA; and assembly and release of the virus. At present, no inhibitors of proviral integration have been developed. However, attention has focused recently on compounds that would inhibit persistently infected cells. One enzyme that appears important in this aspect of viral replication is the viral protease enzyme. Several HIV gene products enhance viral replication, such as the *tat* and *rev* proteins. Inhibitors of these gene products may decrease the number of infectious virions circulating in the body. Finally, the antivirals, such as interferon, which inhibit release of HIV from infected cells, may also offer therapeutic benefit.

Complete inhibition of viral replication by any single drug is a formidable task. Accordingly, antiviral combinations may be more effective than a single antiviral agent alone, especially if the drugs have different mechanisms of action and appear additive or synergistic in vitro in animal models. Studies of combinations of antivirals, such as zidovudine and interferon, zidovudine and CD4, and multiple reverse transcriptase inhibitors, are underway. This latter approach may not only be therapeutically additive, but may decrease the development of in vitro resistance of the virus to these agents, a factor that may be particularly important with reverse transcriptase inhibitors.

The most extensively tested of the antiviral compounds that inhibit HIV in vitro are summarized in Table 11-2. In nearly all in vitro systems, HIV replication resumes when the antiviral drug is removed from HIV-infected cells, indicating that the drugs inhibit productive viral replication, but do not

Table 11-2. Antiviral agents active against HIV in vitro

Agent	Anti-HIV concentration	Achievable serum level	Proposed mechanism of action
Suramin	Suppression at 50 μg/ml; inhibition at 100–1000 μg/ml	>100 μg/ml	Inhibits reverse transcriptase
Ribavirin	Suppression at 10–100 μg/ml	1–3 μg/ml	Inhibits reverse transcriptase
Alpha-interferon	Suppression at 4–64 U/ml; inhibition at 256–1064 U/ml	50–300 U/ml	Inhibits budding
Foscarnet	Suppression at 132 μM; inhibition at 680 μM	100–450 μM	Inhibits reverse transcriptase
Zidovudine	0.13–2.7 μg/ml	0.5–2.0 μg/ml	Inhibits reverse transcriptase; DNA chain termination
ddC	0.1–0.5 μg/ml	0.02–0.04	Inhibits reverse transcriptase; DNA chain termination
ddI	10 μM	0.5–10.0 μM	Inhibits reverse transcriptase; DNA chain termination
Ampligen	Inhibition at 1 μg/ml	NA	Inhibits posttranscript processing, assembly, or release
Soluble CD4	0.3–1.5 μg/ml	NA	Prevents binding
Dextran sulfate (MW 8000)	⩾ 10 μg/ml	NA	Prevents binding

Note: NA = Not available; ddC = dideoxycytidine; ddI = dideoxyinosine.

cure the cell of latently infected provirus. This implies that chronic administration of these drugs will be required. Because HIV is usually present in the central nervous system in most infected persons, antiviral drugs for HIV infection must be able to cross the blood-brain barrier.

Agents that have been shown to potentiate the host's immune system in vitro, such as IL-2, gamma interferon, and levamisol, have been suggested as potential therapies for persons with AIDS and ARC. As single agents, these compounds have shown little utility in patients with advanced HIV infection. It is likely that these agents would need to be used early in the course of infection to be effective. Combination chemotherapy with antiviral agents and these immune modulators may, however, allow these agents to be clinically useful.

CONCEPTS FOR DESIGN AND CONDUCT OF CLINICAL TRIALS

Development of effective animal models for evaluating treatment of HIV infection is a field currently in its infancy. At present, the SIV primate model appears to be the most useful, but preclinical animal studies of antivirals are limited.

Reducing symptoms and opportunistic infections and extending life must be the goals of antiretroviral chemotherapy. Studies designed to foster drug development require large numbers of patients to be followed for extended time periods. Several in vitro criteria have been proposed to evaluate the effects of potential chemotherapeutic agents for HIV in humans. These include decreased ability to isolate virus during and after therapy; improvement of some of the immunologic dysfunctions seen in AIDS, such as an increase in the number of circulating CD4+ cells and restoration of cutaneous hypersensitivity; reversion of other markers of disease production, such as reduction in HIV-1 p24 antigens and beta-2 microglobulin; and a decrease in the clinical manifestations of disease.

ANTIVIRAL AGENTS WITH ACTIVITY AGAINST HIV

Suramin

Suramin, an antiparasitic agent clinically used to treat East African trypanosomiasis and onchocerciasis, was the first drug reported to have in vitro activity against HIV. HIV was inhibited in vitro by a concentration of 100 μg/ml, achievable with a 1-g IV dose. Clinical trials of suramin for HIV treatment began in early 1984. Although isolation of HIV from peripheral blood lymphocytes was transiently decreased, side effects were frequent (including adrenal suppression in 23 percent of patients) and severe, and there was neither clinical or immunologic improvement nor reduction in the frequency of opportunistic infections. This first report of antiviral therapy for HIV illustrated the necessity of controlled clinical trials of antiviral agents for the treatment of AIDS and showed that even well-researched agents may cause adverse clinical effects previously unrecognized in HIV-infected persons.

Ribavirin

Ribavirin is a synthetic purine nucleoside that is active in vitro against a broad spectrum of DNA and RNA viruses, including HIV. It has been widely tested for treatment of influenza A and B and is licensed in the United States in aerosol form for treatment of infection due to respiratory syncytial virus. Oral administration decreases mortality due to infection with lassa fever virus. Ribavirin's mechanism of action is not completely understood, although it is a competitive inhibitor of reverse transcriptase and interferes with viral mRNA synthesis. In vitro, HIV replication is partially suppressed at concentrations of 50–100 μg/ml. Single doses of 600–2400 mg produce peak serum concentrations ranging from 1.2 to 3.0 μg/ml after oral administration and from 10 to 40 μg/ml after IV administration. It has excellent cerebrospinal fluid penetration.

Several trials of ribavirin therapy for HIV have been conducted. However, consistently beneficial results have not been achieved, and most authorities do not believe that it offers much therapeutic benefit. At high doses (greater than 1200 mg per day) it causes lymphopenia. Ribavirin is not licensed for the therapy of HIV-1 infection in the United States or other Western industrialized countries.

Foscarnet

Foscarnet (trisodium phosphonoformate hexahydrate) was first synthesized in 1924 and is structurally related to pyrophosphate. Foscarnet inhibits a wide range of DNA and RNA polymerases, including those of all herpesviruses [herpes simplex virus (HSV), CMV, Epstein-Barr virus, and varicella-zoster virus], hepatitis B virus, and HIV. Foscarnet appears to interact with nucleic acid polymerases at the site where pyrophosphate is released during elongation of the DNA or RNA chain. Foscarnet inhibits HIV reverse transcriptase at concentrations (approximately 1 μM of Foscarnet) that do not affect cell DNA synthesis.

Foscarnet currently is available only as an IV product. It has been tested in humans most extensively as a topical drug for HSV infections and as IV therapy for immunosuppressed patients with severe CMV infection. In the latter studies, a dosage of 20 mg/kg per 24 hours was administered as a continuous infusion. Plasma concentrations ranged from 250 to 500 μM (75–150 μg/ml) during the infusion period. Most of the drug is eliminated unchanged in the urine, with an estimated serum elimination half-life of 6 hours. Foscarnet appears to penetrate the cerebrospinal fluid in patients with and without meningeal inflammation. It appears to offer benefit for CMV retinitis, mucocutaneous HSV infections in acyclovir-resistant mutants, and maintenance therapy for the suppression of CMV infection in immunocompromised patients. Pilot studies with foscarnet as an antiretroviral treatment for patients with AIDS and ARC are underway. Foscarnet does appear to lower serum p24 antigen, but its lack of oral absorption is a major hindrance to its development as an effective antiretroviral.

Zidovudine

Activity and pharmacology. Zidovudine is a clinically effective reverse transcriptase inhibitor of HIV and is marketed under the name Retrovir. Zidovudine is a thymidine analog in which the 3' hydroxy (-OH) group is replaced by an azido (NH_3) group. At concentrations of 0.13 μg/ml or less, zidovudine inhibits 90 percent of detectable HIV replication in vitro. In vivo, zidovudine is converted by cellular enzymes to zidovudine-triphosphate, which is subsequently utilized by HIV reverse transcriptase (Fig. 11-2). When zidovudine-triphosphate is incorporated into the growing DNA chain of HIV, DNA synthesis is terminated.

A series of pharmacokinetic studies of orally administered zidovudine showed that serum concentrations averaged 0.62 μg/ml (range, 0.5–1.46 μg/ml) after chronic oral administration of 250 mg every 4 hours (3–5.4 mg/kg). After oral administration, zidovudine bioavailability is approximately 70 percent due to metabolism in its first pass through the liver. Plasma protein binding is 34–38 percent. Zidovudine's mean terminal half-life is about 1.1 hours. Renal clearance of zidovudine is estimated to be 400 ml/min per 70 kg, approximately 20 percent of total body clearance. The 5'-glucuronide conjugate of zidovudine (glucuronyl-zidovudine) is a major inactive plasma and urinary metabolite. Glucuronyl-zidovudine, with a half-life of approximately 1 hour, is rapidly cleared from plasma. The CSF: plasma concentration ratios vary, but recent studies suggest that most persons receiving 600–1200 mg/per day will have CSF concentrations of 0.028–0.183 μg/ml.

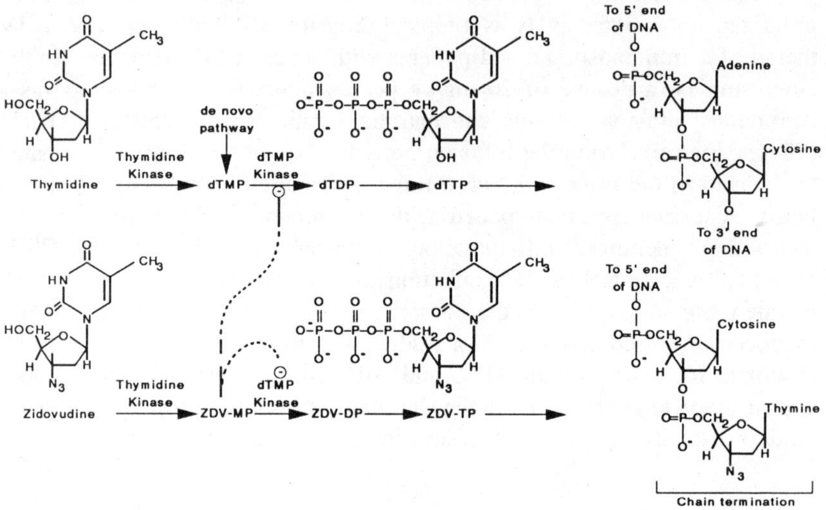

Figure 11-2. The intracellular metabolism of thymidine (top) and zidovudine (ZDV) (bottom). *(a)* ZDV-MP interferes with the phosphorylation of (dTMP) by competitive substrate inhibition. Cells exposed to ZDV may have high levels of dTMP and decreased levels of (dTTP), which may contribute to the drug's toxicity. *(b)* The thymidine pathway at top results in a normal DNA chain. When zidovudine-triphosphate (ZDV-TP) (bottom) is bound by a DNA polymerase and incorporated onto the growing 3' end of a DNA chain, the subsequent 5' → 3' phosphodiester linkages necessary to add other nucleosides cannot form, and the chain is terminated. (Reprinted, with adaptations, by permission from Yarchoan R, Broder S. Development of antiretroviral therapy for the acquired immunodeficiency syndrome and related disorders. *N Engl J Med* 1987;316:561–562.)

Clinical efficacy and toxicity. A phase III, randomized, double-blind, placebo-controlled trial of zidovudine's ability to decrease morbidity and mortality due to AIDS was conducted at 12 U.S. medical centers. A total of 160 patients with AIDS and 121 patients with advanced ARC were studied for an average of 4.5 months. All patients with AIDS recovered from their first episode of PCP diagnosed within the previous 4 months. Patients were given placebo or 250 mg of zidovudine every 4 hours around the clock. Dosages were reduced to 100 mg every 4 hours or permanently discontinued if toxicity developed. After 4 months of therapy, 19 deaths had occurred in the placebo group and 1 in the zidovudine group ($P < .001$). All deaths were due to opportunistic infections or other complications of HIV infection. Because of the decrease in mortality in the zidovudine group, the trial was discontinued for ethical reasons.

In addition to a lower mortality, patients who received zidovudine performed better, functioned better neuropsychiatrically, maintained their body weight, and had fewer and less severe symptoms associated with HIV infection. Preliminary data also suggested some reduction in circulating amounts of HIV core protein (p24) with zidovudine-treated patients. Overall, the 1-year survival rate for patients treated with zidovudine was 80 percent and was higher in some subgroups. Early initiation of therapy was associated with longer survival; survival was highest in those treated early after the onset of PCP and when the CD4 cell counts were higher.

Zidovudine does, however, produce some serious side effects. Granulocytopenia and anemia necessitated dose reduction or drug discontinuation in about one-third of patients (Table 11-3). Blood transfusions were required for about 30 percent of patients receiving zidovudine versus 11 percent for placebo recipients. In general, decreases in hemoglobin and neutrophil levels occur during the second month of therapy and are reversible if the dose is decreased or the drug discontinued. Other side effects reported with zidovudine include rashes, pruritus, nausea, headache, mild confusion, and other neurotoxic symptoms (Table 11-4). Complaints of headache or confusion may precede severe neurotoxicity and should be monitored closely.

Practical guidelines for administration. In March 1987 the FDA approved zidovudine for managing patients with AIDS and advanced ARC who have a history of cytologically confirmed PCP or an absolute CD4 lymphocyte count of less than 200/mm^3 in their peripheral blood. The recommended starting dose is 200 mg orally every 4 hours around the clock, although more recent evidence suggests dosing four times daily; slightly lower dosages are also adequate (see below). Subsequent dosage ad-

Table 11-3. Percent of patients with AIDS and AIDS-related complex receiving zidovudine or placebo who demonstrate hematologic side effects

Hematologic side effect	Zidovudine (N = 113)	Placebo (N = 105)	Zidovudine (N = 30)	Placebo (N = 30)
	Percent of patients			
Granulocytopenia				
<750/mm^3	47	10	10	3
50 percent reduction in baseline value	55	19	40	13
Anemia				
Hgb less than 7.5 g/dl	30	6	3	0
25 percent reduction in baseline value	45	14	10	10

Note: Pretreatment CD4 cell level for zidovudine- and placebo-treated groups was greater than 200/mm^3.

Source: Burroughs Wellcome Retrovir package insert, March 1987.

Table 11-4. Percent of patients with AIDS and ARC receiving either zidovudine or placebo who demonstrate side effects

Side effect	Zidovudine (*N* = 144)	Placebo (*N* = 137)
	Percent of patients	
Headache	42	37
Fever	16	12
Malaise	8	7
Diaphoresis	5	4
Myalgia	8	2
Nausea	46	18
Vomiting	6	3
Diarrhea	12	18
Anorexia	11	8
Gastrointestinal pain	20	19
Dizziness	6	4
Insomnia	5	1
Paresthesia	6	3
Somnolence	8	9

Note: Initial starting dose of zidovudine was 250 mg orally every 4 hours.
Source: Burroughs Wellcome Retrovir package insert, March 1987.

justment should be made as dictated by the toxicity. Most persons feel that dosing four to six times daily is adequate. Hematologic parameters should be carefully monitored at least every 2 weeks; decreases in hemoglobin levels may occur as early as 2–4 weeks, whereas granulocytopenia often is not observed until 6–8 weeks. Recombinant erythropoietin has been used to decrease the frequency of blood transfusions; a treatment investigational new drug status has recently been approved for its use for patients with AIDS on zidovudine who have erythropoietin levels of less than 500 IU.

Zidovudine should be discontinued in patients whose hemoglobin concentration decreases to less than 7.5 g/dl until it is at least 9.5 g/dl. We recommend that patients not be transfused at this time unless their cardiovascular status is compromised or their hemoglobin concentration fails to improve by at least 1 g/dl within 7 days of discontinuing zidovudine. If transfusion is performed, zidovudine may be restarted in 7 days if the hemoglobin concentration has stabilized. In either case, zidovudine should be reinstated at one-half the initial dose (100 mg every 4 hours). If a patient continues to have a low or decreasing hemoglobin concentration, we currently continue the medication if transfusion requirements are less than 4 units every 21 days or if the hemoglobin concentration does not decrease to less than 6.5 g/dl on two consecutive episodes at least 2 weeks apart despite blood transfusions. As described earlier, a trial of recombinant erythropoietin may be useful for patients with decreasing hemoglobin concentrations. If persistent, life-threatening anemia develops (hemoglobin concentration less than 6.5 g/dl), we discontinue zidovudine permanently; this occurs in 10 percent of patients.

Recent evidence suggests that lower doses of zidovudine than those administered in the earlier trials have antiretroviral activity. Recent results from a multicenter trial indicate that 600 mg daily (100 mg six times daily) is as effective as 200 mg six times daily. In addition, patients on lower doses were less neutropenic. We often start patients on 500 – 600 mg of zidovudine daily. If side effects occur, we reduce the dose to 300–400 mg daily. For other severe, zidovudine-induced toxicities, including granulocytopenia (polymorphonuclear leukocyte count = 500–750/mm^3), we discontinue zidovudine until baseline values return. Zidovudine is then restarted at dosages of 300 – 600 mg daily. If severe toxicity resumes, we recommend discontinuing the drug permanently. We currently recommend that the physician confer with a person experienced in the use of zidovudine when toxicity occurs.

Limited information is available regarding the interaction of other drugs with zidovudine (Table 11-5). Coadministration of zidovudine with agents that produce hematologic, nephrotoxic, or cytotoxic effects (dapsone, pentamidine, amphotericin B, flucytosine, vincristine, vinblastine, adriamycin, interferon) may increase the risk of toxicity. All drugs that may competitively inhibit glucuronidation should be used cautiously; these include rifampin, cimetidine, ranitidine, flurazepam, and indomethacin. Acetaminophen has shown little pharmacologic interaction with zidovudine. Probenecid increases zidovudine's half-life and may allow the use of lower doses. Methadone appears to increase zidovudine concentrations; zidovudine doses may need to be reduced if these drugs are used concomitantly. If an opportunistic infection develops, current recommendations are to discontinue zidovudine temporarily, as the chronic administration of many medications with this drug has not been systematically studied. However, if long-term suppressive therapy for an opportunistic infection is required, one should consider using zidovudine concomitantly, with close monitoring for toxicity. Patients taking these medications should be followed by specialists experienced with the clinical presentations of AIDS and the complications of zidovudine therapy.

Use of zidovudine in patients with CD4 cell counts of 500/mm^3 or less. Two recent trials have revealed that zidovudine delays the time to development of ARC in persons who have CD4 cell counts of less than 500/mm^3. In one trial involving patients with early ARC and CD4 cell counts of 200–800/mm^3, participants were randomly assigned to either 1200 mg per day of zidovudine or placebo. After a 9-month (mean) observation period, it was found that zidovudine treatment reduced the frequency of either advanced ARC or full-blown AIDS by 50 percent. Further analysis revealed a significant delay in the progression of disease in patients with CD4 cell counts

Table 11-5. Potential zidovudine drug interactions

Interacting drug	Interaction or mechanism	Clinical significance
Acyclovir	Severe drowsiness and lethargy (two reports); mechanism unknown	None
Dapsone	Increased risk of zidovudine toxicity; additive bone marrow suppression	Avoid concomitant use
Indomethacin	Increased zidovudine or indomethacin toxicity; competitive inhibition of glucuronidation	Avoid concomitant use
Methadone	Increased zidovudine concentrations and possibly toxicity; mechanism unclear	May need to reduce zidovudine dose; interaction under study
Pentamidine	Increased risk of zidovudine toxicity; inhibition of glucuronidation or reduced renal excretion of zidovudine	Avoid concomitant use
Probenecid	Increased zidovudine toxicity; inhibition of glucuronidation or reduced renal excretion of zidovudine	Avoid concomitant use
Ribavirin	Antagonistic antiviral effects	Avoid concomitant use
Trimethoprim-sulfamethoxazole	Increased risk of zidovudine toxicity; zidovudine levels not increased; mechanism unclear	Avoid concomitant use
Vincristine	Increased risk of zidovudine toxicity; additive bone marrow suppression	Avoid concomitant use

below $500/mm^3$. The frequency of developing ARC or AIDS in patients with CD4 cell counts above $500/mm^3$ was too low to indicate any therapeutic benefit. Another study was done with patients who were asymptomatic. In this trial, patients were randomized to groups that received 500 mg per day versus 1500 mg per day of zidovudine or placebo. Approximately 1300 of the 3200 participants had CD4 cell counts below $500/mm^3$ upon entry. Progression to symptomatic HIV disease was evaluated in this latter group. The frequency of developing AIDS was reduced from 6.9 cases per 100 patient years of follow-up in the placebo group compared to 3.9 and 4.2 in the zidovudine groups. Additionally, hematologic toxicity and gastrointestinal complaints were less frequent in patients receiving 500 mg per day of zidovudine compared to those receiving 1500 mg per day. This study strongly suggests that asymptomatic patients with CD4 cell counts below 500/mm^3 should be treated with zidovudine at 500–600 mg per day.

The results of these two studies imply that all HIV-infected persons with CD4 cell counts below 500/mm^3 be treated with zidovudine, and that lower doses are beneficial and less toxic than the 1200 mg daily dose. Although the FDA has not acted on these recent findings, it is expected to do so in 1990. If zidovudine is approved for such use, more than 500,000 people will be eligible to receive zidovudine in an attempt to delay progression of this still lethal disease.

2', 3'-Dideoxycytidine

2',3'-Dideoxycytidine (ddC) is another nucleoside analog similar in structure to zidovudine. It appears to be a more potent inhibitor of HIV replication than is zidovudine. Concentrations of 0.5 μM (0.1 μg/ml) to 2 μM (0.425 μg/ml) inhibit HIV growth and prevent expression of the p24 core protein in T-cell lines. Preliminary data from a phase I trial demonstrated plasma concentrations of 0.02–0.06 μg/ml and 0.2–0.4 μg/ml after single 1-hour IV infusions of 0.03 and 0.25 mg/kg, respectively. The elimination half-life of ddC is approximately 1 hour. It appears to be completely absorbed in both fasting and nonfasting states. CSF penetration has been documented in patients with HIV infection. Patients with AIDS or ARC currently are being enrolled in phase II clinical trials. Side effects observed so far include peripheral neuropathy, a variety of rashes, fever, aphthous stomatitis, thrombocytopenia, and anemia (greater than 20 percent decrease in hemoglobin concentration). The neuropathy appears dose and duration related and appeared after 6–14 weeks of treatment; it resolved several months after ddC was discontinued. A small number of patients have received ddC alternating weekly with zidovudine for a minimum of 6 months. Preliminary results indicate that this alternating regimen is better tolerated at the lower doses than zidovudine alone. Furthermore, sustained elevations in T-cell counts have been observed. Clinical trials comparing ddC with zidovudine are currently in progress.

2', 3'-Dideoxyinosine

2',3'-Dideoxyinosine (ddI) is another nucleoside analog that is a reverse transcriptase inhibitor. ddI is the deamination product of dideoxyadenosine (ddA). Recent phase I clinical trials have shown that at doses of 200–1500 mg per day, ddI has antiretroviral effects. The intracellular half-life of ddA-triphosphate (the active moiety) is longer than that of zidovudine; hence, less frequent (twice daily) administration appears to be needed. Following IV doses of ddI (0.2–3.2 mg/kg), linear increases in peak concentrations were observed ranging from 0.5 to 10 μM, respectively. Of additional importance is detection of ddI in CSF following IV doses. Because ddI is acid labile, oral doses must be administered *after* ingestion of antacids. In this manner, bioavailability averages 35 percent. Early phase I trials in humans suggest that ddI has less hematologic toxicity than does zidovudine. At doses of more than 1200 mg per day, transient neuropathy has been reported. Current phase II clinical trials comparing ddI to zidovudine are underway.

Azdu and D4T

Two additional nucleosides, Azdu (azido-2',3'-dideoxyuridine) and D4T (2',3'-dihydro-2',3'-dideoxythymidine) are currently under development and are entering phase I trials. Their mechanism of action appears similar to that of zidovudine. Less potent in vitro than zidovudine and ddC, they have lower cellular cytotoxicities; hence, their therapeutic indices suggest that they are worthy of clinical testing.

Soluble CD4

As discussed previously, inhibiting HIV attachment by interrupting the interaction between the HIV-gp120 envelope protein and the cell CD4 receptor will inhibit HIV replication. Administering soluble CD4 itself to "flood" the body with CD4 and hence prevent infection of cells is one potential way to accomplish this goal. A recombinant, truncated, soluble CD4 protein has been produced by recombinant DNA techniques in chinese hamster ovary cells. Recent phase I trials have shown that soluble CD4 has minimal toxicity. At doses of 30 mg per day or more, some anti-p24 antigen–lowering effects have been noted. The half-life is unfortunately short; hence, constant administration of high doses appears necessary. Development of a chimeric compound in which CD4 is bound to IgG appears to allow blood levels of CD4 to remain high for prolonged periods. Clinical trials to evaluate the efficacy and clinical effects of long-term administration of these CD4 products are underway.

ANTIVIRAL RESISTANCE

It has recently been shown that stepwise, in vitro resistance of HIV isolates from patients with AIDS treated with zidovudine for extended time periods occurs. The time course for development of in vitro resistance is variable. Although few patients have been studied, the percentage who developed resistance was high. Whether this in vitro resistance correlates with clinical deterioration is, however, not known. Zidovudine-resistant isolates have still been sensitive in vitro to other reverse transcriptase inhibitors, such as ddC and ddI, but have been resistant to Azdu. These data have spurred the concept of using combinations of antiretrovirals or other reverse transcriptase inhibitors. However, it is not clear how frequently disease progression during zidovudine therapy is due to resistance to the drug or progressive replication of the virus from chronically infected cells not inhibited by a reverse transcriptase inhibitor.

OTHER AGENTS

Castanospermine is a glycosylation inhibitor that exhibits an anti-HIV effect by altering the envelope glycoprotein of HIV (a heavily glycosylated protein). The drug appears to inhibit lymphocyte syncytium formation by the virus and, therefore, may slow the depletion of T4 cells, which may be due to syncytium formation. Preclinical testing of an analog called *N*-butyldeoxynojirimycin is underway.

Ampligen, a polynucleotide derivative of poly I-poly C, is mismatched, double-stranded RNA that protects lymphoblastoid cells from HIV infection in vitro. Although it is effective in vitro, early phase I testing has shown little overall antiviral effect.

INTERFERONS

Several interferon preparations have been evaluated in patients with AIDS, especially those with AIDS and Kaposi's sarcoma. Recombinant interferons have been shown to have an effect against both HIV and Kaposi's sarcoma; however, these antiviral and antitumor effects are only partial. The antiretroviral effect of interferons is not as great as that of anti-reverse transcriptase inhibitors. As both alpha-interferon and zidovudine decrease granulocyte counts, they appear to have enhanced toxicity; however, these compounds also exhibit in vitro synergy. Studies are underway to define a maximally effective dosage regimen.

COMBINATIONS OF ANTIRETROVIRALS

Several combinations of antivirals have demonstrated additive, synergistic, or antagonistic effects on inhibition of HIV. Studies suggest that combinations of drugs may have enhanced clinical efficacy and may inhibit HIV replication at better-tolerated levels and more easily achieved concentrations in vivo. Additionally, such combinations may prevent the selection of drug-resistant HIV mutants. Presently, however, no evidence supports correlations between in vitro synergy and enhanced clinical outcome.

Interactions between zidovudine and interferon and between zidovudine and the antiviral agent acyclovir have stimulated interest in HIV combination therapy. In vitro, both drugs enhance zidovudine's inhibition of HIV. The mechanism of acyclovir-zidovudine synergism is unknown; however, because acyclovir is a well-tolerated drug with no hematologic toxicity, its use with zidovudine warrants investigation. Alpha-interferon prevents the release of infectious viruses and, hence, inhibits HIV at a different stage in the viral replication process than does zidovudine. The AIDS Clinical Trials Group program of the National Institutes of Health has begun phase II trials with this combination. Additionally, foscarnet, ddC, and lymphoblastoid interferon have been found to be synergistic with zidovudine in vitro.

Not all antivirals have additive or synergistic effects, as illustrated by the in vitro antagonistic effects between zidovudine and ribavirin. Ribavirin appears to increase deoxythymidine-triphosphate levels, which causes feedback inhibition of thymidine kinase. This reduces phosphorylation of zidovudine to zidovudine-triphosphate. These data also suggest that ribavirin should not be used in vivo with zidovudine or similar derivatives, except under investigational conditions. The clinical importance of the in vitro antagonism of zidovudine and ribavirin requires clarification. On a more positive note, ribavirin is synergistic in vitro with foscarnet.

TREATING THE HIV-INFECTED PATIENT WITH ANTIRETROVIRAL AGENTS

Currently, there are several avenues through which an HIV-infected patient may receive antiretroviral therapy. These include FDA-approved agents, study protocols governed by the National Institutes of Health, and study protocols governed by the investigative pharmaceutical industry. Recently, another program for selective distribution of drugs through an expanded access and compassionate-use system has been developed.

Because zidovudine is the only FDA-approved agent, all physicians can prescribe zidovudine for such patients. However, information is lacking on the efficacy and safety of zidovudine for HIV-infected patients who are asymptomatic and have high CD4 cell counts. Several large, controlled studies of persons in the earlier stages of HIV infection are underway. The benefits and risks of zidovudine for these patients are unknown. It is conceivable that the early administration of zidovudine will actually be deleterious over the long term in asymptomatically infected patients.

Congress has appropriated money for persons who meet the package-insert requirements to receive zidovudine. Reimbursement for zidovudine is available for some low-income persons who lack Medicaid assistance, third-party medical insurance with prescription drug coverage, or income in excess of 185 percent of the national poverty level. To apply for support in most states, the prescribing physician and patient must complete an eligibility application form. This form, along with the name and address of the dispensing pharmacy, must be sent to the appropriate state agency.

SUMMARY

The field of antiviral chemotherapy for HIV infection is rapidly developing. Many new potential therapeutic approaches are under investigation. As of this writing, zidovudine is the only FDA-approved agent that has been shown to be clinically effective. Zidovudine use currently is restricted to patients who have overt AIDS or symptomatic ARC with fewer than 200 circulating CD4 cells/mm^3. Zidovudine toxicities, including neutropenia and anemia, are significant. Careful monitoring of hematologic parameters is essential when using zidovudine, and dose reduction and occasional discontinuance of the drug may be necessary. Coadministration of other drugs, such as probenecid or trimethoprim-sulfamethoxazole, should be done with utmost caution. Because zidovudine is not a cure for HIV infection, and because HIV appears to be a lifelong infection requiring chronic treatment, studies are underway to enhance zidovudine's clinical benefit. While the search for more efficacious and less toxic treatments continues, the prolongation of life that zidovudine has shown provides hope that further progress in this area will continue at its present rapid pace.

ADDITIONAL READING

Fischl MA, Richman DD, Grieco MH, Gottleib MS, Volberding PA, et al. The efficacy of azidothymidine (AZT) in the treatment of patients with AIDS and AIDS-related complex. *N Engl J Med* 1986;317:185–191.

Francis DP, Petricciani JC. The prospects for and pathways toward a vaccine for AIDS. *N Engl J Med* 1985;313:1586–1590.

Hirsch M, Kaplan JC. Treatment of human immunodeficiency virus infections. *Antimicrob Agents and Chemother* 1987;839–884.

Mitsuya H, Broder S. Strategies for antiviral therapy in AIDS. *Nature* 1987;325:773–778.

Richman DD, Andrews J. Results of continued monitoring of participants in the placebo-controlled trial of zidovudine for serious human immunodeficiency virus infection. *Am J Med* 1988;85(suppl 2A):208–213.

Richman DD, Fischl MA, Grieco MH, et al. The toxicity of azidothymidine (AZT) in the treatment of patients with AIDS and AIDS-related complex. *N Engl J Med* 1987;317:192–197.

Vogt M, Hirsch MS. Prospects for the prevention and therapy of infections with human immunodeficiency virus. *Rev Infect Dis* 1986;8:991–1000.

Yarchoan R, Broder S. Development of antiretroviral therapy for the acquired immunodeficiency syndrome and related disorders. *N Engl J Med* 1987;316:561–562.

12

Psychosocial Aspects of HIV Infection and AIDS

Terence C. Gayle
Lewayne D. Gilchrist
Heather Andersen

Primary care physicians will be involved increasingly in the direct care of patients with HIV disorders ranging from asymptomatic, HIV-antibody seropositivity to overt AIDS. The physical conditions of such patients are inextricably bound to their individual psychological processes, as well as to the reactions of the people around them. Physicians must recognize the psychosocial component of suffering and how psychological and social issues contribute to the disease process and provision of care. Awareness of these issues is essential to the integrity of the physician-patient relationship and to fulfillment of the oldest and most important goal of the profession—to relieve suffering, regardless of the chances for cure. Accomplishing this goal requires frank discussion about fears surrounding the disease, treatment options, risk reduction, and referral to a variety of mental health and social service resources when appropriate.

At least three realities complicate physicians' ability to care for patients with AIDS-related diseases. The first is our constantly changing understanding of the pathophysiology of HIV infection. AIDS-related diseases are varied and sometimes difficult to identify, and their courses are often unpredictable. The prognosis is often uncertain. Statistics regarding prevalence, prognosis, and modes of transmission often do not answer the questions and address the concerns of the individual patient.

The second reality is that most persons at highest risk for AIDS are members of stigmatized social groups. Identifying a patient's actual risk status requires taking a careful history of sexual behavior and patterns of illicit drug use. Physicians usually have little training in this area and may be reluctant to question patients directly on these topics.

The third reality is the usual need to coordinate aspects of care for HIV-infected patients with other care providers in the community. Out-of-hospital care for debilitated patients with AIDS or other advanced HIV-related infections may require the cooperation of one or more social service agencies. The crushing emotional reactions of many patients, plus the necessity to help patients make lasting changes in sexual behavior, may require referral to psychiatrists and other mental health professionals. Many physicians are unaware of such resources in their communities, and some communities lack such resources altogether.

In this chapter, we illustrate psychosocial issues as they relate to five groups of patients. The first three groups include: persons with AIDS; those with symptomatic HIV infection without overt AIDS; and asymptomatic, seropositive people. The other two groups include the "worried-well," high-risk persons who thus far are seronegative; and persons at low risk who are seronegative but are nevertheless concerned about their health. Patients in each of these groups face clinically relevant psychological, social, and behavioral issues.

ISSUES RELATED TO OVERT AIDS

In many ways, reactions to AIDS are similar to those seen in patients with cancer and other life-threatening illnesses. We can examine the process of coping with catastrophic illness in a framework of three phases of adaptation. The process begins with initial awareness of the threat, proceeds through a transitional period of active integration of limitations into daily life, and usually ends in a new state of psychic equilibrium marked by an acceptance of the imposed limitations.

The notion of stages of adaptation is offered here as a general guideline only. Actual movement through these phases is often neither linear nor orderly. Rather than progressing to an ultimate resolution, a person may recycle through the set of phases with each subsequent adverse event, such as a decline in health status. This framework is relevant to clinical care because it can help the clinician make an optimal match between an intervention and the patient's stage of adaptation.

Acute crisis phase

Persons with newly diagnosed AIDS typically experience an initial crisis marked by waves of extreme anxiety which alternate between denial and emotional numbness. The initial shock of the diagnosis may be less in persons who already suspect that they have AIDS because of a recent gradual decline in health status. In this first phase, persons with AIDS may be too overwhelmed to remember many details of the medical information presented. The best therapeutic stance is to provide emotional support, answer repeated questions as honestly as possible without taking away hope, and acknowledge that intense emotions are part of a normal stress response syndrome. An example of an honest yet supportive statement to a patient with newly diagnosed Kaposi's sarcoma might be "You have Kaposi's sarcoma. So far, the average life expectancy for someone with this disease is about 2 years, but some people with AIDS have had Kaposi's sarcoma for several years and are still living productive lives. Research on antiviral drugs and other treatment for AIDS is moving quickly. With good nutrition, stress management, rest, regular exercise, and avoidance of new infections, you could help keep the virus from gaining an even bigger foothold and from progressing as rapidly." The initial crisis phase can last for periods ranging from days to several weeks and corresponds roughly to the period of the first hospitalization or the first few weeks after outpatient diagnosis of AIDS.

Shortly after the diagnosis is confirmed, patients are confronted with a barrage of questions and decisions, such as whom to inform, who else may be at risk, what to tell employers, how to handle changes in finances and home arrangements, and how to evaluate treatment options. In this stage, most persons with AIDS will benefit from a crisis intervention approach that reinforces previous psychological strengths and breaks the wall of difficult problems into smaller pieces that can be managed one at a time. The patient needs to know that hasty decisions are not necessary and that time is available to deal with most of these issues.

A certain amount of denial is adaptive in the early stages. However, too strong a persistent denial of the diagnosis and its implications can lead to noncompliance with medical care or failure to make necessary practical decisions. Because social support is critical, involvement of the person's significant other or closest friend in discussions and plans is essential to enhance coping.

Transitional phase

After the initial crisis resolves, patients with AIDS enter a middle, or transitional, phase. During this period, the patient struggles with two tasks: coping with the practical problems of daily living in the face of increasing disability and anticipatory grieving over future losses. Existential issues related to the meaning of one's life, along with fears of death and dying, become paramount. AIDS is particularly isolating because it is associated with such highly politically and emotionally charged issues as homosexuality, presumed sexual promiscuity, drug use, fear of contagion, and death. Fear of loneliness and abandonment can be eased by scheduling regular follow-up appointments with a consistent primary care physician, referring persons to AIDS support groups or individual counselors, and linking them with volunteer "buddies" or companions.

Physical contact—a massage or merely an empathetic hand on the shoulder—often provides a sense of comfort and cuts through feelings of isolation and loneliness (Fig. 12-1). Because many persons with AIDS have known others who died of the disease, their fears of pain and suffering are realistic. Gruesome expectations may be ameliorated by early discussion of palliative treatment for pain and other symptoms. To sustain hope and to counter fears of dependency and loss of control, it is vital that the person retain as much autonomy as is permitted by the physical condition. Most patients need to participate as equal partners in all management decisions.

Home care is more humane than prolonged hospitalization and usually is

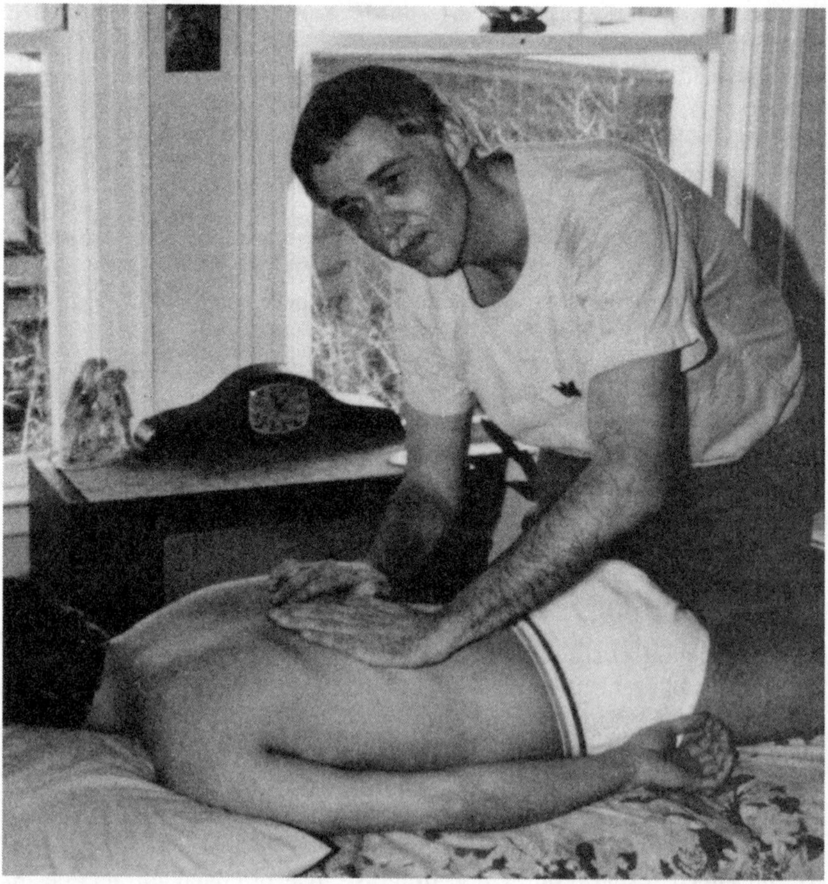

Figure 12-1. Seattle massage therapist Bob Fuller donates his time to work with patients with AIDS.

more cost-effective. As disability increases, chore care services can help keep the person at home longer. If the person's sense of identity is closely bound to a job, then encouragement to return to the job or to participate in volunteer work can help fend off the fear of loss of identity. Fear of disfigurement, especially common in young persons concerned about body image, can often be lessened by empathetic statements that reinforce the intrinsic worth and good of the person, regardless of emaciation, cutaneous lesions, or other external manifestations.

Persons with AIDS describe an emotional roller coaster in response to changes brought on by the disease. A resurgence of hopelessness is most likely to occur at times of treatment failure or subsequent rehospitalization. The personal meaning of the disease for the patient with AIDS is often the source of much suffering. Rumination over the question "Why me?" frequently leads to guilt about sexual orientation, past sexual partners, or other lifestyle factors. We cannot overemphasize the importance of helping to alleviate this guilt to reduce the burden of suffering. Persons with AIDS need to be reminded that they have the disease not because of who they are but because they are infected with an impersonal virus.

Most persons with AIDS will admit to thoughts about suicide. Sometimes the idea seems to represent a somewhat comforting symbol of self-determination and destiny in the face of so much that is uncontrollable. Negotiable environmental changes—for example, housing, assistance with chores, and companionship—can sometimes dramatically reduce suicidal intent, as can counseling about relationship problems. The incidence of suicide in patients with AIDS is not well defined, but the experience of the gay community on the West Coast suggests that suicide is relatively infrequent, albeit not negligible.

The recent availability of zidovudine has provided a source of hope for persons with AIDS, but also may create additional complexities for patients trying to make decisions about treatment and the future. They must weigh the benefits of prolonged life against zidovudine's high cost and the possibility of drug intolerance or the need for frequent transfusions. One of the most gratifying benefits of this drug may be its ability to reverse or at least halt the AIDS dementia syndrome (see Chap. 11).

Persons with AIDS often experience dramatic realignments of the spiritual and philosophical aspects of their lives. The adaptive focus on the quality of their remaining time may result in a new, positive spirit that can have a powerful effect on friends and caregivers. It is crucial that the physician be tolerant and supportive of a patient's religious conversion, for example.

One issue that sometimes surfaces is the compatibility of traditional medical care with alternative treatments. This issue has surfaced more frequently since the evolution of organizations in many cities that provide information about both traditional and alternative therapies for AIDS. A patient's active search for alternatives can be an important part of coping and should not be discouraged immediately. Patient-physician agreements on concurrent strategies, whereby the physician is informed of alternative treatments and informs the patient of any potential harm are possible. Most alternative therapies are not harmful if they do not replace standard care.

A significant proportion of patients suffer the additional burden of AIDS dementia complex, major depression, and other psychiatric disorders associated with medical illness (see Chap. 8). In particular, major depression is suggested by prolonged loss of self-esteem, unremitting guilt, and the inability to experience pleasure in anything. Because of the high probability of eventual cognitive dysfunction, persons with AIDS should be strongly encouraged to take an active part in getting their affairs in order as early as possible after diagnosis. This includes completing a will, designating a durable power of attorney, and making funeral arrangements. These activities actually promote a sense of personal control. Cardiorespiratory resuscitation status and the patient's desires concerning intensive care (e.g., intubation) should be determined within the first 72 hours of each hospitalization.

Terminal phase

The terminal phase typically occupies the final days or weeks before death. During this time, the patient with AIDS turns inward and retreats from the world. Because family and loved ones may feel rejected, it is helpful to interpret this phase for them as part of the natural death cycle, thus giving the patient permission to withdraw. The dying person may feel the need to complete unfinished personal business with loved ones. In this phase, the caregiver's principal goal is to facilitate a death that is as free of pain and isolation as possible. During all phases, persons with AIDS are especially subject to social isolation imposed by some hospital infection-control procedures and the avoidance behaviors of some health care workers. Such isolation can be lessened by explaining necessary precautions to the patient and by acknowledging and confronting our own fears of AIDS and our attitudes toward members of high-risk groups and ethnic minorities with disproportionately high rates of HIV infection.

The following case example points out one of the most important aspects of care for patients with AIDS: the need for a multidisciplinary team approach. Caring for persons with AIDS is difficult, even with access to the best resources. No one primary care clinician can possibly provide all facets of care required. We strongly urge case management with orchestration of a variety of services to provide efficient, quality care and to prevent provider burnout.

CASE 1: AIDS

John is a 32-year-old gay man. He was diagnosed as having ARC a year before his first episode of PCP. His local support system includes a lover of 3 years and several friends. He was successfully employed as a bookkeeper at an insurance company but had to quit his job 6 months ago because of difficulties with routine arithmetic, caused by slow but progressive cognitive dysfunction.

Acute crisis phase

- John's lover is included in discussions of a treatment plan.
- John's physician asks if John wants his parents to know that he has AIDS and whether they know he is gay.
- John is referred to a community support group so that he can establish a relationship with a volunteer before discharge.

Transitional phase

- John's physician schedules twice-monthly follow-up appointments, refers John to a weekly AIDS support group, and refers John and his lover to a therapist for joint counseling regarding interpersonal conflicts resulting from the strain of AIDS.
- With the help of a case-management agency and a group of volunteer lawyers who work with persons who have AIDS, John completes his will and arranges for his lover to have durable power of attorney if John becomes mentally incapacitated.
- John decides that he does not want to be intubated if he has another episode of PCP.
- When John begins to appear depressed, withdraws socially, and has more memory complaints, he is referred to a psychiatrist, who diagnoses major depression and begins antidepressant treatment; the depression improves, but the cognitive dysfunction worsens.
- The psychiatrist asks John's volunteer team to place signs around John's house as memory aids (e.g., "Turn off the stove.")
- As John develops motor problems, a chore care worker comes in to help with cleaning, cooking, and bathing.

- John's lover is referred to a support group for partners and families of persons with AIDS to vent his grief over John's declining health.

Terminal phase

- As John becomes moribund, his physician and social worker conduct a family conference that includes John's parents and lover; they sort out individual responsibilities that make everyone feel useful.
- John dies in the company of his lover, having previously completed unfinished business with his family.
- Memorial services are conducted according to John's wishes.

ISSUES RELATED TO SYMPTOMATIC HIV INFECTION WITHOUT AIDS

Research has consistently indicated that HIV-infected patients with mild to moderate symptoms experience higher overall levels of emotional distress than persons with AIDS. Anxiety is the most prevalent mood disturbance. This is not surprising if one realizes that symptomatic patients without AIDS live in a purgatory of prognostic uncertainty. Prolonged anxiety may eventually give way to depression. Many of these patients are keenly interested in their doctor's opinions of ways to prevent progression to AIDS, such as antiviral chemotherapy, prophylaxis for opportunistic infections, diet, vitamin use, and other possible measures. One way to deal with the uncertainty is to shift the perspective from concern about eventual death to living in the present. Some patients undergo the same philosophical and spiritual development as do those with AIDS. Relaxation training and positive imagery often are effective in reducing anxiety and should be tried before prescribing benzodiazepines unless the anxiety is functionally disabling.

Because of self-imposed isolation and the frequent lack (in most geographic areas) of focused resources for symptomatic persons without AIDS, helping them find a support system is one of the best things a physician can do. Patients can benefit greatly from participation in support groups. Referral for couple counseling is indicated when symptomatic HIV infection disrupts the patient's interpersonal relationships or causes problems in communication.

One should keep in mind that symptomatic patients with AIDS also have an increased risk of developing such neuropsychiatric problems as cognitive dysfunction and major depression. In Case 1, John showed signs of an insidious dementia that led to work impairment well before AIDS was diagnosed.

ISSUES RELATED TO ASYMPTOMATIC HIV INFECTION

For many persons, confirmation of their seropositive status comes as a surprise, even when they appear intellectually prepared for that possibility. Such confirmation can be acutely distressing. Irrefutable proof of infection can quite suddenly bring with it the specter of lifelong disability, disease, lost or irreparably changed sexual expression, and death—all of which most young, physically well persons are ill-prepared to confront. Although experience is still limited, zidovudine treatment may ameliorate these stresses in some patients (see Chap. 11).

CASE 2: ASYMPTOMATIC HIV INFECTION

Roy, a 29-year-old gay man, recently ended a 3-year relationship when his partner, Mark, left for a new job in a distant city. Roy and Mark had a mutually monogamous relationship. Although he and Mark had never used condoms, Roy had never worried about HIV infection or AIDS. Anxious about reentering the dating scene and managing new sexual relationships, he decides, somewhat impulsively, to be tested for HIV antibody. Disclosing his verified negative status to prospective partners will be advantageous, he thinks, and his seronegativity will give him an incentive to adhere to safer sex and other health-affirming practices.

Although appropriately counseled prior to testing, Ray gave no real thought to the possibility that he might be seropositive. News of his seropositive status devastated him. He subsequently realized that although he knew that he and Mark had had a mutually monogamous relationship, he knew very little about Mark's life and sexual partners before they met.

Acute crisis phase

- Give Roy time to absorb the news and to ventilate anger and other negative feelings.
- Avoid attempts at complex problem solving or clinical instruction during the period of maximum emotional upset.
- Reassure Roy, if necessary, that he will not infect friends through casual contact.

- Begin clinical assessment (medical history, physical examination, blood and skin tests); reassure Roy that the preliminary examination is normal (if appropriate).
- Schedule a follow-up visit in a few days to continue medical evaluation and emotional support.

Acceptance phase

- Perform a complete medical evaluation; discussion of the prognosis and the ability to affect it favorably (zidovudine, other prophylactic therapy) may contribute substantially to emotional support.
- Give Roy safer sex guidelines and discuss any problems he foresees in putting the guidelines into practice.
- Refer him to a support group for seropositive men.
- Plan with Roy how and when he will tell Mark about his HIV status and how Roy can advise Mark to be tested.
- Discuss case reporting, if in a state with a reporting requirement.
- If needed, refer Roy to a psychotherapist for help with anger at his ex-partner and with changing to safer sex.
- Advise Roy regarding eating properly, avoiding infection, and other health and lifestyle issues.

Following confirmation of their seropositive status, most patients want to know their chance of developing AIDS or other serious symptoms. The data from recent longitudinal studies of seropositive gay men and hemophiliacs are sobering; up to 75 percent develop significant symptoms or AIDS over 10 years (see Chaps. 7 and 8). However, it seems likely that these statistics will improve as antiretroviral chemotherapy and treatment to prevent opportunistic infections are increasingly developed and employed. Even with such treatments, the gravity of the possibility of developing AIDS, coupled with the prognostic uncertainty, can lead to frustration for both physician and patient. Many seropositive patients want advice about diet, exercise, and other health-affirming activities to help them feel more in control of their health. Many want explicit information about how modes of virus transmission may affect their typical activities. They ask such questions as "What kinds of casual contact are safe?" "Can I kiss my mother without worrying that I will harm her?" "How much at risk is my partner?" "Can I ever have sex again?"

Table 12-1 outlines accepted prevention guidelines (see also Chap. 3). Physicians may be called upon to translate these general guidelines into

Table 12-1. Categories of behavior relative to the risk of HIV infection

	Behaviors	
	Sexual	**Parenteral drug use**
Safe	Sexual abstinence Noninsertive sexual relations: hugging, kissing (if oral lesions not present), genital manipulation (if no skin lesions present) Social (dry) kissing Body-to-body rubbing ("frottage") Fantasy, masturbation	Abstaining from drug use Avoiding injection with used equipment
Possibly safe	Vaginal intercourse with condom and spermicide French kissing (wet) External contact with body fluids (e.g., skin contact with urine, saliva, or semen) Fellatio, without intraoral ejaculation Cunnilingus	Disinfecting shared injection equipment with bleach
Not safe	Analingus (rimming) Fisting (inserting fingers or hands in rectum) Any contact involving blood Sharing insertive sex toys (e.g., dildos) Semen or urine in mouth Anal insertive intercourse* Vaginal intercourse without a condom	Using injection equipment used by another person

Note: In counseling, use of the patient's own terminology for safer sex practices is more effective than use of medical terminology.

*Although condoms and spermicides reduce the risk of HIV transmission by anal intercourse, the risk of condom rupture may be substantial; anal intercourse should be considered risky even if a condom is used.

explicit everyday behavior in clear, unmistakable terms. Although transmission-prevention guidelines seem clear, they can be extraordinarily difficult to put into practice. For example, intellectual commitment to using condoms at every sexual encounter can quickly break down when negotiating condom use with a partner one doesn't want to alienate or when judgment is impaired by sexual excitement, alcohol, or other drugs. Among some groups of IV drug users, a culture of sharing needles exists that is difficult to avoid without dissociating from the group entirely. If the group provides a person's only social support, such dissociation may be extremely difficult. Where compliance with transmission-prevention guidelines may be especially difficult, it may be helpful to refer the patient to a psychiatrist, psychologist, social worker, or other behavioral specialist.

Research suggests that a simple and effective way to assess probable compliance is to ask the patient in a nonjudgmental way, "Do you think you will be able to use a condom every time you have intercourse, or do you think you will probably not be able to arrange this?" If the patient anticipates trouble, ask, "Would you like to be referred for counseling to teach you how to do it?" Many local health departments and AIDS support agencies can help with referral for such counseling.

Newly diagnosed seropositive patients usually have many concerns about the confidentiality of their test results. Patients may have serious (and, in some cases, realistic) worries that they will lose their jobs or health insurance if their status is disclosed to an employer or an insurer. Physicians, clinics, and hospitals treating HIV-infected patients need to consider how they will deal with these important issues of confidentiality (see Chap. 3). Legal counsel regarding such matters may be helpful.

Seropositive patients in sexual or needle-sharing relationships have a clear obligation to inform their partners of their HIV-positive status. Physicians can help patients plan this disclosure and should strongly suggest that patients' partners voluntarily undergo serologic testing and receive counseling about infection control. A disturbing ethical dilemma is thought by some to arise when a physician knows that a seropositive patient is continuing unprotected, high-risk sexual activities or sharing needles with an uninformed partner. Although the duty to warn those at risk may be at odds with the professional commitment to confidentiality, there is broad agreement that the duty to protect an unsuspecting partner must take precedence. In some states, this obligation is codified in law (see Chap. 3). Physicians who treat seropositive patients should examine their own values and consider what actions they will take if confronted with this dilemma.

ISSUES RELATED TO SERONEGATIVE DIAGNOSIS: THE "WORRIED-WELL"

Patients in this category fall into two groups: those whose past or current behavior clearly places them at risk of infection and those whose past and current behavior makes infection unlikely or highly improbable. Physicians should be knowledgeable about the pros and cons of the HIV antibody test in this setting. To assess the advisability of testing a patient, physicians should take a history thorough enough to assess the patient's risk status realistically (see Chap. 6). Many health care providers do not routinely ask patients about sexual behavior or about drug use and possible needle sharing. If physicians assume a patient's risk status without taking a structured history that focuses on specific high-risk behaviors, they can misjudge the patient's true vulnerability.

TAKING A SEXUAL HISTORY

The key to taking a successful sexual history is the clinician's acceptance of sexuality as an important aspect of the patient's overall health. This is much easier if the physician feels comfortable with his or her own sexuality. People are sensitive to verbal and nonverbal cues of willingness to discuss sexuality and will be much more open to such discussion if they perceive that the physician is accepting and nonjudgmental.

Early questions should be open-ended and make use of the term *partner(s)* instead of *he* or *she*. Rather than asking direct questions about sexual orientation, men and women can be asked: "Do you have sex with men, women, or both?" The subsequent questions should try to establish whether the patient is having sex with a steady partner, for how long, and whether there is sex with persons of either gender outside the primary relationship. Questions about frequency and type of sexual practices (oral, anal, vaginal, etc.), number and types of contacts (e.g., anonymous), locations of sex acts, and consistency of preventive measures or safer sex (i.e., use of condoms, spermicides, or abstention from unsafe sex) will yield essential information for assessing relative risk status for AIDS and STDs.

Other important items include when the last sexual exposure with steady or other partners occurred, the patient's STD history, and whether any partners have symptoms of STDs or are otherwise at risk for HIV infection. It is better to use explicit and graphic anatomic terms and the patient's own terms for sexual practices, because not all patients will understand terms such as *insertive* or *receptive oral sex, fellatio,* or *cunnilingus*. One could ask instead, "Do you take his penis in your mouth?" Some people make distinctions between "having sex," "making love," and "fooling around," and unsafe sex may be included in some or all of these designations. Among different ethnic cultural minority groups, there are different terms for sexual practices, as well as different ways of thinking of and labeling one's own sexual orientation.

Throughout the interview, if one senses that the patient is having difficulty talking about sexual issues, it is helpful for the clinician to acknowledge this difficulty openly while stressing the importance of this discussion in the overall medical evaluation. Once rapport is developed, the patient is generally more willing to hear the physician's concerns about certain activities and suggestions for behavioral change that will reduce risk. Of course, similar issues concerning the use of vernacular language and a nonjudgmental attitude and approach also apply when taking a history concerning illicit drug use.

CASE 3: HIGH-RISK, SERONEGATIVE PATIENT

Stan, age 29, has been married for 4 years and has a satisfying sexual relationship with his wife. Stan's job requires extensive travel. During his travels—without his wife's knowledge—Stan has unprotected anal intercourse with men he meets in gay bars. Although Stan knows that he may be risking infection and placing his wife at risk as well, he has not considered antibody testing. He feels certain that if his wife or his employer knew of his homosexual activities, he would lose everything.

During a routine physical examination, Stan casually remarks that AIDS affects only "flaming queers." His physician says that HIV infection occurs because of certain behaviors, regardless of sexual orientation. Stan's distressed reaction leads his physician to ask pointed questions about high-risk behavior. Stan and his physician agree that he should be tested for HIV infection. Stan is told that if he is seropositive, his wife (and other identifiable sexual partners) must be notified. Although this frightens him and generates considerable discussion, Stan recognizes that his wife's health is paramount.

Stan's test shows him to be seronegative. He tells his physician that he wants to stay that way but isn't sure that he can control his sexual behavior.

- Listen carefully for underlying true concerns.
- Obtain a sexual history that is sufficiently complete to assess Stan's real risk status.
- Allay Stan's fears regarding the confidentiality of antibody test results.
- Assess Stan's ability to cope with possible confirmation of seropositive status; make sure that he fully understands the nature of the test and its consequences, or refer him to someone who can do this pretest counseling.
- Do an antibody test or refer Stan for testing; advise him to have additional tests 3 and 6 months after his last high-risk exposure to avoid the possibility that he has been infected but has not yet seroconverted.

- Give Stan clear guidelines on safer sex practices.
- Provide him with references for counseling or mental health resources to help him achieve lasting behavior change in order to reduce his risk of infection.

Stan's apparently satisfactory relationship with his wife could lead to the assumption of exclusive heterosexuality and, therefore, low-risk status. One should inquire directly whether the patient has engaged in unprotected anal intercourse since 1978, especially as a receptive partner, or has shared needles since that time. Most patients who have engaged in high-risk behavior will not volunteer this information until asked directly in a nonjudgmental manner. Fewer than one-third of homosexual men disclose their sexual orientation to their physicians unless queried directly in the context of AIDS risk assessment.

Patients like Stan may benefit from counseling to help them change long-standing behavior that puts them at risk for infection. Making changes in behavior patterns is not easy; changing sexual and drug-using behavior may be especially difficult. Physicians should have available a list of referral resources—local self-help groups, psychiatrists, other mental health professionals in private practice, or counseling and mental health agencies—to help the patient achieve lasting, protective behavior change.

Finally, some patients' psychological makeup leads to irrational fears that they have or will get AIDS. Discomfort with sexuality in general, guilt over perceived past indiscretions, and a host of other psychological reasons can lead to acute worry or even panic among patients who have little real risk of infection. Media attention to the AIDS epidemic clearly has contributed to such irrational fears.

CASE 4: LOW-RISK, SERONEGATIVE PATIENT

Roger, age 49, is a divorced, heterosexual, white man who comes in with concerns that he may have AIDS. He had sex with a prostitute once in 1962. A complete sexual, drug, and medical history and physical exam reveal that he has no other risk for HIV infection and is in apparently good physical health. He constantly checks himself in the mirror, looking for further symptoms of AIDS and is worried about such things as normal "shoddy" inguinal lymph nodes, long-standing moles, fatigue, initial insomnia, and what he thinks is a persistent "coating on the tongue." He also reveals that he has been tested for antibody to HIV at least 15 times over the past 3 years. He has seen several other doctors but has been dissatisfied because their workups failed to reveal any organic disease. Despite consistently negative results and reassurance, his anxiety about AIDS persists and is interfering with his personal and social life.

The coping stages presented earlier are not relevant to this situation. Somatization can present as a feature of several primary psychiatric disorders. Such patients often become disappointed or angry if they are told that "the problem is in your head." They tend to refuse psychiatric referral and continue shopping for doctors or alternative providers in their quest for an explanation of and treatment for their illnesses. It is important that somatizing or hypochondriacal patients be screened by the primary care physician for such treatable psychiatric disorders as major depression, panic or other anxiety disorders, obsessive-compulsive disorders, psychotic disorders, and substance abuse, as well as the more difficult to treat primary hypochondriasis and somatization disorder. Malingering related to AIDS occurs but is rare.

If the patient's behavior is part of an entrenched somatizing style, the best approach is to maintain the physician-patient relationship by scheduling regular appointments, avoiding costly medical workups and unwarranted surgical procedures, and admitting one's limitation in being able to come up with a disease or a "magic bullet." By listening to the patient's somatic preoccupations and then asking how these are affecting his or her life and mood over many sessions, the physician can strengthen the relationship, diffuse anger and frustration, identify psychosocial stressors and triggers, and allow the patient to ventilate emotions in a way that is more acceptable than as a "mental patient." Such patients should be kept out of AIDS support groups and other activities that might reinforce their identity as a sick person. They can benefit from involvement in other social groups and activities, especially if they are unemployed, bored, lonely, and have a limited social support network. Over time, some may eventually accept psychotherapy.

Medical personnel can use their authority and credibility to reassure patients such as Roger that the risk of HIV infection is negligible and that testing is unnecessary. If reassurance proves insufficient, testing may be warranted, despite the small risk of false-positive or indeterminate results that could exacerbate the patient's distress (see Chap. 6). Whether or not the test is done, referral for counseling and mental health care—perhaps in addition to serologic testing—may alleviate the patient's anguish.

ADDITIONAL READING

Cohen MA, Weisman HW. A biopsychosocial approach to AIDS. *Psychosomatics* 1986;27:245–249.

Faulstich ME. Psychiatric aspects of AIDS. *Am J Psych* 1987;144:551–556.

Holland JC, Tross S. The psychosocial and neuropsychiatric sequelae of the acquired immunodeficiency syndrome and related disorders. *Ann Intern Med* 1985;103:760–764.

McKusick L, Horstman W, Abrams D, Coates TJ. The psychological impact of AIDS on primary care physicians. *West J Med* 1986;144:751–752.

Nichols SE. Psychosocial reactions of persons with the acquired immunodeficiency syndrome. *Ann Intern Med* 1985;103:765–767.

Perry S, Jacobsen P. Neuropsychiatric manifestations of AIDS-spectrum disorders. *Hosp Comm Psych* 1986;37:135–142.

Wolcott DL, Namir S, Fawzy F, et al. Illness concerns, attitudes towards homosexuality, and social support in gay men with AIDS. *Gen Hosp Psych* 1986;8:395–403.

13

Perspectives of a Primary Care Physician on Managing Patients with AIDS

Julia R. Smith

As an internist, I have provided primary care in the last 4 years to more than 70 patients with various stages of HIV infection—from asymptomatic to end-stage AIDS. The issue of AIDS has even touched some of my established patients who are at low risk for HIV infection. Some have requested testing to ease fears of "a casual encounter a few years ago"; a neighbor wanted to advise her 16-year-old daughter about kissing. My involvement with AIDS and related conditions has challenged me more than any other condition I have encountered to engage the science, the art, and the politics of medicine.

THE SCIENCE OF AIDS: INFORMATION AVAILABLE BUT SKETCHY

As a rule, physicians are most comfortable when grounded in the science of medicine. The science of AIDS, however, is evolving so rapidly that we are often uncertain about what we have to offer. There is more information than any generalist can keep up with. Although specific information is readily available by telephone from publicly funded AIDS projects (see Chap. 16) and from specialist consultants, the following case illustrates key questions that remain difficult to answer.

CASE 1

Karen is a health professional. Following the normal delivery of her first child, she learned that she had been transfused with HIV-positive blood 2 years earlier. Her newborn was seropositive, reflecting maternal antibody or perinatal infection.

In trying to counsel Karen about the risks to her neonate, it would be possible to offer retrovirus cultures of the newborn's blood. (Positive culture would indicate infection of the newborn, but sensitivity of culture in this setting is uncertain.) The risk of perinatal transmission is still uncertain, and the prognosis for the perinatally infected infant is not yet well-defined. In counseling Karen about her own risks of AIDS, the prognosis for an otherwise healthy young woman infected by transfusion is quite variable.

AIDS IS THE PROVINCE OF PRIMARY CARE

Because of the specialized nature of information on AIDS and its complications, one might consider the disease a subspecialty problem. For several reasons, I believe that the management of persons with AIDS and related conditions falls most naturally into the province of primary care medicine. Many of our patients are concerned and request information about AIDS. AIDS must now be considered in the differential diagnosis of many illnesses. It affects multiple organ systems and thus requires input from several subspecialties, rather than falling solely within the province of any single specialty. Primary care providers can best coordinate the advice of consultants, as well as the case management of many psychosocial problems.

We all must be prepared to answer questions about AIDS and to clarify for patients what they learn from the media or hear in casual conversation. Health maintenance screening of all sexually active persons should routinely include questioning about risk factors and education about protective sexual practices. Many of us will see asymptomatic, antibody-positive persons who will benefit from the usual primary care screening and advice. However, such patients need emotional support in the midst of the uncertainties about their conditions, as well as continuity with a physician who can evaluate symptoms and problems as they arise.

Appropriately evaluating symptoms in antibody-positive individuals with Group I or Group II disease is a major clinical challenge to the primary care provider (see Chap. 8). When does one suspect PCP in the patient with cough, cerebral toxoplasmosis in someone with headache, or treatable intestinal infection in someone with loose stools? How exhaustively should one work up fever, fatigue, or nausea? HIV-infected persons can experience viral bronchitis or gastroenteritis, migraine headache, or excessive stress. Considerations that dictate a careful search for opportunistic infection are illustrated by the following case.

CASE 2

Richard is a 33-year-old, married, seropositive, bisexual man with a history of fatigue and frequent bouts of axillary hydradenitis. He developed a fever of 103° F and myalgia without respiratory symptoms. The physical examination was unremarkable, and the illness subsided in 5 days. High fevers returned 3 weeks later, along with a mild, dry, cough. The chest x-ray was clear, but the arterial blood pO_2 was 70. Pulmonary diffusion capacity was significantly reduced, and subsequent bronchoalveolar lavage showed *Pneumocystis carinii*. He received sulfamethoxazole-trimethoprim for 1 week, developed nausea and vomiting, was switched to pentamidine for 2 more weeks, and is doing well 2 months later.

The duration and severity of the illness are helpful in evaluating common symptoms. The presence of features of more common illnesses—rhinitis, a typical pattern for tension headache, or irritable bowel, or isolation of common pathogens—may help to identify a more benign condition. Clinical evidence that suggests deterioration of the patient's immune function—such as onset of oral thrush or prolonged outbreaks of herpes—might raise suspicion about opportunistic infections. Similarly, decline of the total lymphocyte count or CD4 lymphocyte count is associated with an increased risk of such infections; PCP is uncommon in HIV-infected individuals with CD4 cell counts greater than $200/mm^3$. Unfortunately, CD4 cell counts were not available at the time of presentation in the above-described case. In deciding when to pursue more extensive workup, physicians may want to consider the treatability of a potential AIDS-related disease. Clinicians must deal with the patient's need for reassurance in deciding how to interpret various symptoms. A telephone call to a subspecialist about the extent and timing of workup may be helpful.

COORDINATING SUBSPECIALTY CARE

When symptoms unique to AIDS develop, a subspecialist often is needed to assist in diagnosis and in planning therapy. However, the continued central involvement of the primary care provider is most important. Serial problems involving multiple organ systems may require several consultants. The generalist plays the pivotal role in coordinating management, ensuring continuity, and assessing various subjective considerations in determining a treatment plan. The following cases illustrate issues in coordinating subspecialty care, in withholding invasive diagnostic studies, and in withdrawing therapy.

CASE 3

Stephen is a married, bisexual man with AIDS that had presented as blurred vision due to CMV retinitis. After ophthalmologic evaluation, he was placed on an antiviral drug, ganciclovir, which his wife administered IV at home. He developed an unsteady gait and uncontrolled movements of his arm. Cerebrospinal fluid protein was slightly elevated. The CT scan was unremarkable, but severe nausea and vomiting led to an MR imaging scan that showed several lesions in the cerebellum suggestive of infection. Despite treatment for presumptive toxoplasmosis, follow-up MR imaging showed possible progression of the lesions. Infectious disease and neurology consultants suggested brain biopsy as the only way to identify any potentially treatable disease. Stephen and his wife conferred with me before electing to forego biopsy and receive home terminal care.

The couple felt that the potential benefits of finding the cause of only his most recent symptoms would not be worth the additional risks, discomfort, and added hospital time for brain biopsy.

CASE 4

John was a 39-year-old gay man who had been treated for PCP. He developed persistent diarrhea; special examinations of the stool revealed only cryptosporidia. Because opiates failed to control the diarrhea, we administered the experimental drug spiramycin, without response. After 2 months of worsening symptoms, John was rehospitalized for IV hyperalimentation and for fluid and electrolyte replacement. Endoscopy and small bowel biopsy by a gastroenterologist revealed no curable causes for the diarrhea. Anticipating death, John arranged for a friend to assume legal guardianship. After being hospitalized for 4 months and requiring 6 to 8 liters of fluid replacement a day, John requested that the IV support be discontinued. The orders were written, and he was allowed to die.

Since this experience, I have avoided prolonged hospitalization for other patients with AIDS by arranging 24-hour nursing care at home, providing supplemental nursing or hospice support to other care providers in the home, or arranging alternative residential placement where nursing or other support is available. In many instances, private insurers will fund such arrangements.

To assist the patient or family in choosing between aggressive treatment in the hospital versus home therapy, or between continued efforts to prolong life versus comfort measures to support the dying process, we must be familiar with the psychosocial and spiritual elements of the situation as well as with the biomedical (see Chap. 12).

THE ART OF CARING FOR PERSONS WITH AIDS

The personal involvement required in the art of caring for persons with AIDS includes the physician's acceptance, emotional support, and willingness to face the issues of death and dying with these patients, and an openness to learning from them. A prerequisite is to deal honestly with our own fears and denial and with the inevitable sense of helplessness that comes when we have no more science to offer.

For many patients with AIDS, the illness provides an occasion for self-examination, reestablishing priorities of values, and completing unfinished business in their lives. Despite the fatal prognosis, a tremendous amount of healing can occur in persons with AIDS and in those around them.

If the traditional definition of health refers only to the absence of physical disease, then healing is no longer possible for those with HIV-related conditions. But the healing that occurs for many persons with AIDS is a sense of wholeness (the root word of *health*) that results from accepting and integrating all the facets of oneself, even in the face of disability and death. Technology in this setting takes on a new purpose: to give the patient more time for healing and to minimize suffering. Our task as primary care providers is to facilitate this process by recognizing its importance, providing emotional support (often just by listening), and arranging psychosocial assistance when needed.

PRACTICAL MATTERS: COORDINATING PSYCHOSOCIAL SUPPORT

Coordinating all available psychosocial services is the practical side to the art of caring for persons with AIDS. While we tend to focus on the mechanics of patient care in the hospital or office, patients spend most of their time at home. There they discover various functional limitations and face the full trauma of their diagnosis.

It is beyond our capacity as private practitioners to handle all psychosocial issues. In large cities there may be hospital- and community-based services to oversee such matters. Much work also may be done by volunteers, often from the city's gay and lesbian communities. Even so, greater participation and support from the public at large will be essential to meet the needs of the growing population of persons with AIDS (see Chap. 3). City governments need to develop housing and skilled nursing facilities for patients with AIDS and to make home care assistance more available. Physicians' involvement in lobbying for such services could have great impact on the quality of life available to their patients.

In smaller communities, services must be created by modifying or expanding existing systems. Groups such as the American Red Cross, home care services, community college departments of social work, and the religious community may already provide resources that can serve patients with AIDS. Support from businesses and the media can have tremendous influence in developing needed community systems and services. Neighbors, friends, and volunteers can act as caseworkers to access these services where a formal system is not developed. Medical professionals need to be active at the outset in smaller communities to lobby, inform, and guide community and service agencies in providing adequate care.

COMMUNITY SERVICE AND THE POLITICS OF AIDS

Employing the art of medicine may involve us in the politics of medicine as well. With AIDS, such involvement seems unavoidable. As a physician, I personally feel a responsibility to participate in public education about AIDS and to help dissipate public fear and paranoia about the disease. As long as there is ignorance and fear of the modes of HIV transmission, we face the risk of discriminatory and ineffective public policy decisions. We can no longer associate this disease with a few stigmatized social groups. It is important to understand the virus and its potential effect on us all. Our ability to meet the needs of HIV-infected persons and to educate our populace effectively about preventive measures will only be as great as our acceptance of AIDS as a community problem.

As physicians, we are regarded as sources of authoritative information in such matters. We have an opportunity and a responsibility to take the lead in influencing and shaping public policy regarding AIDS, thereby affecting the course of this epidemic in our society.

14

Infection Control in AIDS and HIV Infection

Patricia Lynch
Walter E. Stamm

Since the onset of the AIDS epidemic, nosocomial transmission of HIV to health care workers has been a major concern. As of January 1990, fewer than 20 hospital-based health care workers and one dentist in the United States reportedly had acquired HIV infection in the course of their work. None has developed AIDS. Nosocomial transmission of HIV to other patients or visitors has been neither reported nor suspected in any health care setting. These data clearly indicate that the risk of nosocomial HIV transmission is low. Nonetheless, health care workers are understandably concerned (and sometimes fearful) about their personal risk and are universally eager to employ whatever infection-prevention strategies might be effective for themselves, patients, and visitors. Some of the major questions regarding nosocomial infections and AIDS include the following:

- Are health care workers likely to become infected by caring for patients with AIDS, and if so, how?
- Are health care workers likely to become infected with the opportunistic infections characteristic of AIDS patients?
- Are patients likely to become infected when cared for by a health care worker with HIV infection?
- What circumstances might lead to indirect transmission of HIV through the use of shared equipment?
- Are other patients (particularly roommates) or visitors at risk for nosocomial transmission of HIV or opportunistic infections?

Although direct answers to all of these questions are not yet available, the risks of HIV transmission in the hospital and possible prevention strategies are becoming increasingly clear. We review them here.

THE PARALLEL WITH HEPATITIS B VIRAL INFECTION

In the early 1980s, several studies confirmed what anecdotes had long suggested: health care workers in some occupational categories are much more likely to have serologic evidence of hepatitis B virus (HBV) infection than is a more representative population, such as volunteer blood donors. Occupational exposure to blood was identified as the major risk factor associated with HBV acquisition in health care workers. Thus, the highest rates of HBV infection were observed in emergency ward nurses, pathologists, dentists, laboratory staff, and surgeons. Lower rates were observed in ward nurses and medical house staff. Patients also acquired HBV from infected health care workers under some circumstances, usually during invasive procedures such as surgery or dentistry. Occasionally, inadequately disinfected equipment—for example, endoscopes or dialysis machines—appeared to play a role in HBV transmission.

Like HBV, HIV is present in blood and other body secretions such as semen and, in lesser quantities, in saliva and urine. Both viruses also are transmitted through sexual and blood contact. Thus, it is easy to understand why health care workers are concerned about nosocomial HIV acquisition. If HIV and HBV are transmitted by the same routes, and if the same infection-prevention strategies that have been relatively unsuccessful for HBV are used for HIV, the risk of HIV transmission would seem substantial.

Although these two diseases share the same routes of transmission, they do not appear to be spread with equal ease. After a needlestick exposure to an infected patient's blood, the risk of HBV transmission is 25–30 percent, while the risk of HIV transmission is less than 1 percent. A partial explanation for this difference may be that the blood of HIV-infected persons appears to have far fewer infectious particles than does the blood of a person infected with HBV, reducing the likelihood of transmission from an average inoculum. Other virus and host factors, as yet undefined, are also undoubtedly important.

RISK OF HIV TRANSMISSION FROM AN INFECTED PATIENT TO HEALTH CARE WORKERS

Several prospective studies have now reported the results of monitoring more than 2000 hospital personnel for HIV acquisition after needlestick injuries or mucous membrane exposures to known AIDS patients. In a study conducted by the CDC between 1983 and 1988, 3 (0.5 percent) of 860 hospital employees seroconverted after needlestick or other sharp injury exposure to the blood of HIV-infected patients. No seroconversions were seen among 103 personnel who had mucous membrane rather than sharp injury exposure to blood. Other prospective studies at individual hospitals have produced similar results, leading to the conclusions that infection occurs in 0.5–1.0 percent of those exposed to HIV-positive blood by needlestick or other penetrating injury and that infection is extremely low after nonblood exposures or after exposures to blood that do not involve penetrating injuries. Outside of prospective studies, there have been, as of January 1990, case reports of at least 14 health care workers in whom nosocomial HIV infection is believed to have occurred, and all had occupational exposure to blood. Nine of the health care workers were punctured with contaminated needles or other sharp instruments; two of these persons were inadvertently injected with small volumes of the patients' blood. In one case, spattered blood was ingested, and in two cases, broken skin may have played a role in acquisition. Several of the patients involved were not known to have AIDS when the health care worker was exposed.

Since the epidemic began, more than 100,000 people in the United States have met the definition of AIDS. Most of those patients have been hospitalized at least once, generating hundreds of thousands of patient-caregiver contacts. Except for the cases mentioned previously, no transmission to personnel, visitors, or other patients has been documented. No cases of HIV infection have been suspected or proved to be related to nonsexual or non-blood-related contact, including bites from infected patients. In a large study of household contacts of AIDS patients, no HIV infection was transmitted even though some household members shared the patients' razors and toothbrushes (see Chap. 1).

TRANSMISSION OF OPPORTUNISTIC INFECTIONS

Patients with AIDS develop frequent and recurrent opportunistic infections (see Chap. 8). The severity of these illnesses makes hospital personnel question whether the infectious agents are particularly virulent or readily transmissible within the hospital. In fact, most infections in patients with AIDS are opportunistic pathogens that infect only individuals with inadequate immune function. Thus, the risk to healthy hospital employees of infection with *Pneumocystis carinii, Mycobacterium avium intracellulare, Toxoplasma gondii,* or *Cryptococcus neoformans* is negligible. Other pathogens that commonly cause opportunistic infections in patients with AIDS—including herpes simplex virus, varicella-zoster virus, *Candida,* and

CMV—already have infected many normal individuals. In patients with AIDS, such infections recrudesce and disseminate; in persons with a healthy immune system, they remain dormant.

Although no cases of opportunistic infections in patients, visitors, or health care workers associated with patients with AIDS have been reported, three infections commonly seen in these patients could cause nosocomial infections in health care workers. Patients with AIDS are at increased risk for tuberculosis, and hospitals that care for these patients should routinely give personnel tuberculin tests. Hospitals also should place patients with tuberculosis in private rooms and use approved ventilation systems to reduce the transmission risk. Transmission of herpes simplex virus or varicella-zoster virus from extensive mucocutaneous lesions to health care workers' unprotected fingers can produce herpetic whitlow, and nosocomial transmission of varicella-zoster virus to a nonimune adult could lead to severe varicella infection. All health care workers dealing with such skin lesions should wear gloves.

PRECAUTIONS TO PREVENT NOSOCOMIAL TRANSMISSION OF HIV AND OPPORTUNISTIC INFECTIONS

What precautions are reasonable, and for whom should they be used?

Several news stories have highlighted the issue of precautions to prevent HIV transmission. In Washington, D.C., police assisting with traffic and crowd control wore rubber gloves when working near the hotel where the Third International AIDS Conference was held. In New York, jurors and court attendants wore masks and rubber gloves while a man with AIDS was on trial. Garbage collectors in Boston refused to pick up trash from the local AIDS Project office. In a fairly large survey of house staff, respondents thought that they were at risk for acquiring AIDS and should be allowed to refuse to care for patients with AIDS. Appropriate infection precautions must be aimed at preventing known avenues of transmission, but educating personnel to eliminate unfounded fears is also of great importance (Fig. 14-1).

Traditionally, hospitals have focused on using precautions for known cases of disease. This approach presumes that most infective cases can be readily recognized and diagnosed. Unfortunately, this is not true of AIDS or of many other infectious diseases. For this reason, the concept of identifying known cases and then taking extra precautions with just those cases may

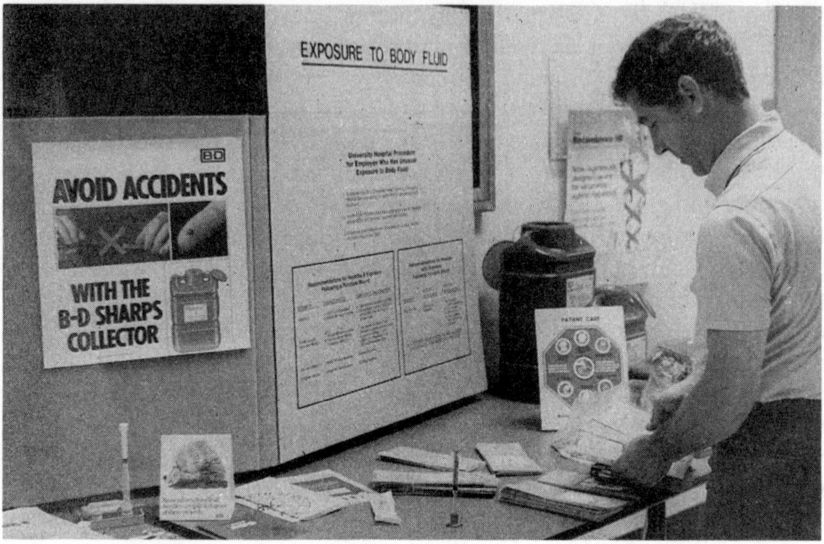

Figure 14-1. University of Washington Hospital employees learn about the appropriate use and disposal of sharp medical instruments during Sharps Awareness Week.

lead to a false sense of security and to relaxation of precautions with other patients, and thus may facilitate transmission from unrecognized cases.

SCREENING FOR HIV AS A BASIS FOR PRECAUTIONS

The issue of screening patients for HIV infection upon hospital admission continues to generate debate. The San Francisco AIDS Task Force discussed the value of screening *all* hospital patients for HIV and concluded that it is preferable to use infection precautions for contact with blood and body substances from all patients. This approach improves the overall standard of care and ensures that precautions are not relaxed for patients with negative test results who might later be infectious. Additional disadvantages of screening include its considerable expense, low yield, and occasional false-negative and false-positive results. The CDC also suggests that the strategy of using precautions with all patients be followed in dental offices and when performing invasive procedures. Others have advocated preoperative screening for HIV, especially when it is not feasible or economically practical to take maximal precautions for every procedure.

A GENERIC APPROACH TO INFECTION CONTROL: BODY SUBSTANCE ISOLATION

Since HIV infections often go clinically unrecognized, precautions taken just with blood and body substances of individuals known to be infected will not adequately protect personnel. Instead, precautions must be taken with all patients. At Harborview Medical Center in Seattle, this strategy has been used exclusively since 1985. The key elements of the system, called *body substance isolation,* are as follows:

- Wear gloves when contact with blood, mucous membranes, nonintact skin, or moist body substances is likely.
- Wash hands before patient contact and whenever (despite gloving) soiling occurs.
- Wear gowns or plastic aprons when it is likely that health care worker's clothing will be soiled by moist body substances from any patient.
- Wear masks, goggles, glasses, hair covers, or other barriers as necessary to protect personnel from splashing or soiling.
- Use private rooms for patients who extensively soil the room with moist body substances or who have airborne communicable diseases. Patients with AIDS do not routinely need private rooms.
- Place all used sharps—needles or other instruments capable of cutting or puncturing—in rigid containers and autoclave them before disposal (Fig. 14-2).
- Handle trash and soiled linen from all patients uniformly. Put heavily soiled linen through a cold-water rinse cycle before washing. Bag trash securely and dispose of it in keeping with facility policy and regulatory agency requirements.
- Handle all laboratory specimens as if the patient were known to be infective.

Every patient room has a sign outlining these precautions (Fig. 14-3). For patients with communicable diseases that can be transmitted by air, an additional room sign requests check-in at the nurses' station before entering so that susceptible persons can be kept out. To help keep the patient's diagnosis confidential, signs do not identify the patient's disease and precautions do not depend on diagnosis (except with airborne communicable diseases).

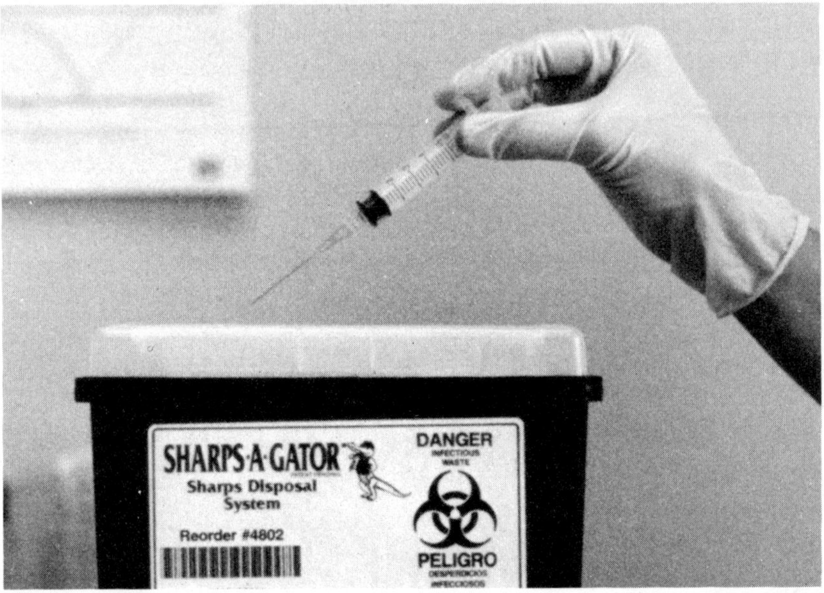

Figure 14-2. To avoid the risk of needlestick transmission of HIV, used needles should not be capped or manipulated before disposal in a puncture-resistant container. (Photograph by Doug Arditti.)

This system of precautions offers substantial protection to personnel but is a major change from the diagnosis-dependent isolation systems that many hospitals have used for years. Personnel need to wear gloves more frequently, creating a challenge to inspire physicians and other health care workers to comply. In general, our medical staff has accepted this system as easy to understand because the rationale is clear and easy to implement because it eliminates many of the categories and category-specific practices of previous systems.

INEFFECTIVE PRACTICES

Gowns, masks, gloves, or other protective barriers are not needed unless contact with a patient's mucous membranes, nonintact skin, blood, or moist body substances is likely. Excessive use should be discouraged. The use of disposable plates and eating utensils is not beneficial and gives patients cold, unattractive meals. Protective isolation—as practiced in general hospitals—neither prolongs life nor decreases the number of infections in compromised hosts such as patients with AIDS.

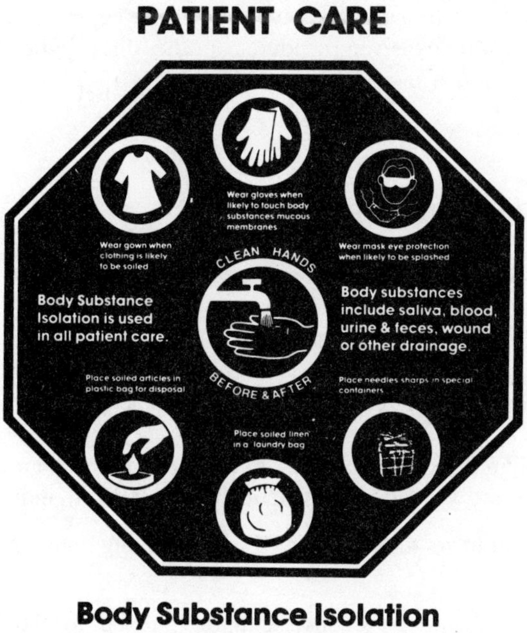

Figure 14-3. This poster, developed at Seattle's Harborview Medical Center, reminds hospital staff about body substance isolation procedures for all patients.

PRECAUTIONS FOR SPECIAL CIRCUMSTANCES

Invasive procedures include all surgical, dental, obstetric, and other procedures that involve entry into tissues, cavities, or organs. Except for one possible case reported in a dentist, no cases of HIV transmission from a patient to a health care worker or from a health care worker to a patient during an invasive procedure have been reported. The following precautions are recommended.

- Health care workers must wear gloves when touching mucous membranes or nonintact skin of all patients and must use other barriers when indicated (e.g., masks and goggles if body fluids are likely to be aerosolized). Gloves should be changed between patients and when glove punctures or tears occur.

- After use, disposable syringes and needles, scalpels, and other sharps must be placed in puncture-resistant containers. Needles should not be recapped or manipulated. Techniques that minimize penetrating injury due to scalpels, surgical needles, and so forth must be used in all operative procedures.

- No health care worker with exudative lesions or weeping dermatitis should perform or assist in invasive procedures or other direct patient-care activity or handle equipment used for patient care.

EXPOSURE MANAGEMENT

Health care workers with parenteral or mucous membrane exposure to patients' blood should report the incident to the appropriate hospital department. Similarly, if a patient has parenteral or mucous membrane exposure to a health care workers's blood, the patient should be told of the incident. Subsequent management recommendations are the same for both groups.

- The donor source should be identified and informed. The recipient should be evaluated and treated prophylactically for HBV if indicated.
- The donor should be screened for HIV after giving consent and receiving counseling.
- The recipient should be counseled and screened for HIV as soon as possible after the incident to establish baseline information. Recipients found to be HIV positive need not be screened again. Recipients who are serologically negative should be screened again at 3, 6, and 12 months after the incident. Seroconversion usually occurs within 3 months. The effectiveness of administering zidovudine to the recipient after exposure is unknown and is currently under study. The decision as to whether to provide 6 weeks of zidovudine to a recipient after an exposure should be made on an individual, case-by-case basis after considering the type of exposure, the stage of the patient's disease, and other factors.

LABORATORY PRACTICES

Laboratory personnel should adhere to P2-level containment procedures for all specimens. This involves wearing gloves when the hands are likely to be soiled with any specimen, wearing lab coats or disposable gowns when clothing is likely to be soiled, and using other barriers such as masks and goggles when aerosolization is likely (Fig. 14-4). Mouth pipetting, smoking, and eating at the benches is prohibited. Blood spills are cleaned by gloved personnel using a disinfectant approved as tuberculocidal.

Many hospitals use biohazard labels for blood or other specimens being

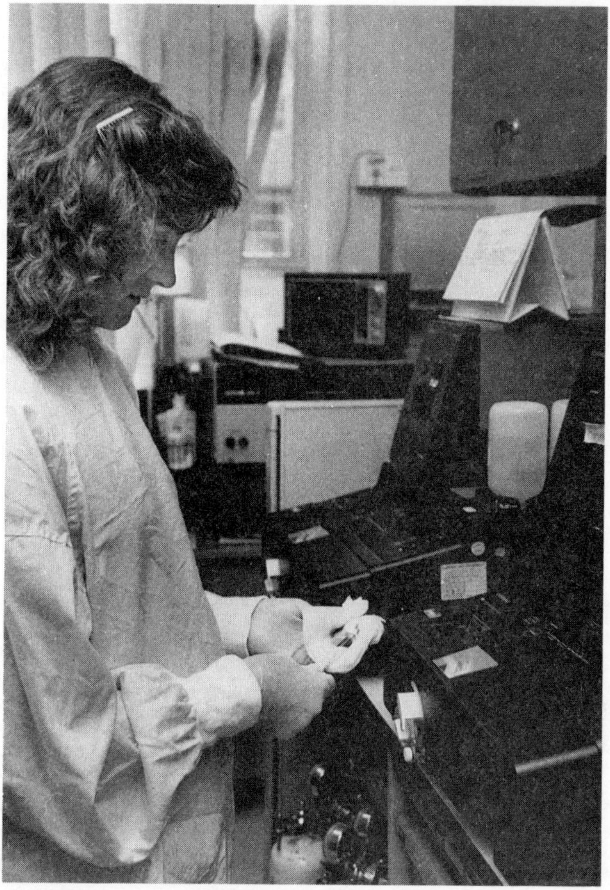

Figure 14-4. Debra Mantyla, a medical technologist in the chemistry laboratory at Harborview Medical Center in Seattle, is gloved and gowned in accordance with P2-level containment procedures.

sent to the laboratory from patients with AIDS, HBV, or other infections. This policy has the same shortcomings as disease-specific isolation precautions: because many infections are not clinically apparent, lables are not affixed to all potentially infectious specimens. The high rate of HBV transmission in laboratory workers may reflect in part the failure of such labeling practices. In our view, all specimens entering the laboratory must be considered potentially infectious and should be handled with appropriate precautions.

RESUSCITATION

Mechanical resuscitation equipment (Ambu bags) should be readily available in all health care facilities. No cases of seroconversion following oral resuscitation of an HIV-infected patient have been reported, but use of mechanical equipment is preferable.

HEALTH CARE WORKERS WITH HIV INFECTION

Health care workers infected with HBV occasionally have transmitted the infection to patients, usually while performing invasive procedures. This phenomenon has not yet been reported with AIDS and probably is less likely to occur, but it seems prudent that health care workers with HIV infection avoid participating in invasive procedures. Routine patient care probably can be safely provided by HIV-seropositive health care workers who are otherwise healthy and do not have open lesions.

SUMMARY

Current data sugest that a health care worker's risk of HIV infection from an infected patient is small but certainly present. Needlestick injuries or other direct exposures to blood from HIV-positive patients account for the cases reported to date, and preventive measures to reduce the occurrence of these specific events are of great importance. Casual contact does not result in HIV transmission from patients to health care workers, and most opportunistic infections of AIDS patients pose little risk to health care workers. Health care workers should use appropriate precautions for anticipated contacts with the blood or secretions of any hospitalized patient, not just those with AIDS or any other infection.

ADDITIONAL READING

Centers for Disease Control. AIDS and HIV update: Acquired immunodeficiency syndrome and HIV infection among health-care workers. *MMWR* 1988;37:229–234.

Centers for Disease Control. Recommendations for prevention of HIV transmission in health-care settings. *MMWR* 1987;36(2):1S–19S.

Centers for Disease Control. Recommended infection control practices for dentistry. *MMWR* 1986;35:237–242.

Centers for Disease Control. Update: Universal precautions for prevention of transmission of HIV, hepatitis B virus, and other bloodborne pathogens in health care settings. *MMWR* 1988;37:377–382.

Dienstag JL, Ryan KM. Occupational exposure to hepatitis B virus in hospital personnel: Infection or immunization. *Am J Epidemiol* 1982;115:26–39.

Gerberding JL, Henderson DK. Design of rational infection control policies for HIV infection. *J Infect Dis* 1987;156:861–864.

Gerberding JL. Recommended infection control policies for patients with human immunodeficiency virus infection: An update. *N Engl J Med* 1986;315:1562–1564.

Klein RS, Phelan JA, Freeman K, et al. Low occupational risk of human immunodeficiency virus infection among dental professionals. *N Engl J Med* 1988;318:85–90.

Lynch P, Jackson MM, Cummings MJ, Stamm WE. Rethinking the role of isolation practices in preventing nosocomial infections. *Ann Intern Med* 1987;107:243–246.

15

The Duty to Treat Patients with AIDS

Albert R. Jonsen

Is it ethically permissible for a physician to refuse to treat a patient with AIDS or one who has positive test results for HIV antibody?

U.S. law does not require physicians to provide services to any particular patient unless a special relationship already exists. The Principles of Ethics of the American Medical Association (AMA) state that a physician may choose those whom he or she wishes to serve.[1] In the United States, there has long been a reluctance to force one person to provide services to another against his or her will. Thus, it would appear that no physician has either a professional or a legal obligation to treat a patient with AIDS.

However, the role of the physician in our culture has long been identified with a willingness to serve those in need at a cost or danger to self. Although history records instances in which physicians abandoned the sick to save themselves, there is a long record of selfless service, particularly in the epidemics of cholera, yellow fever, influenza, and polio that ravaged the

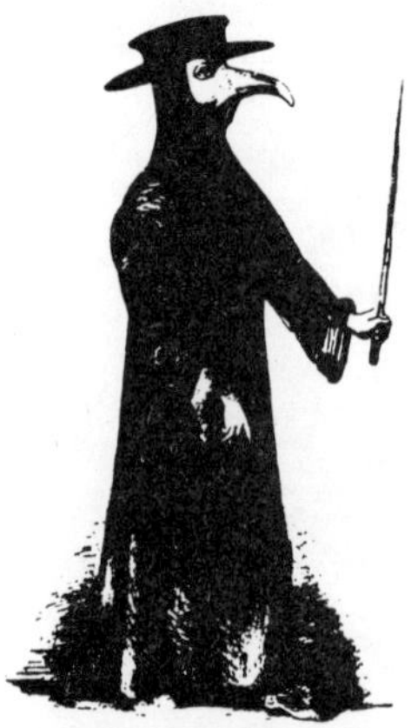

This physician is dressed in the garb worn during the bubonic plague epidemics in Italy in the 1600s. The heavy cloak functioned as a "body glove" to ward off the alleged atmospheric poisons believed to spread plague. Because people also believed that such poisons leaked through the skin and were exhaled in breath, the spice-filled beak was relied upon as an air purifier and the wood stick made it possible to take a pulse without touch.

United States in the last century and in the first half of this century. This record has been an important ingredient in the positive reputation of medicine and of physicians.[2]

So important was this ingredient that the AMA compromised its strong stand in favor of the rights of the physician by making an exception in time of epidemic. The original version of its Code of Ethics (1847) contained the following passage: ". . . when pestilence prevails, it is their [the physicians'] duty to face the danger and to continue their labors for the alleviation of suffering, even at jeopardy to their own lives."[3] That passage was eliminated in 1957, when the threat of epidemics seemed over, but when AIDS appeared, the Judicial Council of the AMA reaffirmed the physician's duty: "A physician may not ethically refuse to treat a patient whose condition is within the physician's realm of competence . . . neither those who have the disease [AIDS] nor those who have been infected with the virus should be subject to discrimination based on fear or prejudice, least of all by members of the health care community."[4] Almost all major organizations of physicians and providers have issued similar statements.

Still, statements of professional organizations, however solemn, do not themselves create an ethical principle. These statements must rest on an ethical principle independent of the contingent preferences and politics of their members. Does such an ethical principle exist? If it does, how strictly must it be observed? Are there circumstances in which a physician may refuse to respond to a person's need without being considered unethical?

The principle would require that a person's medical need establishes his or her moral claim on the attention of persons with medical training. In the recent literature on the subject of professional responsibility, philosophers, physicians, and historians have examined the grounds for such a principle. Some have found it in the traditions of the profession, others in the nature and character of the physician's role, and still others in the reciprocal obligations between society and the profession. Regardless of the form of the argument, almost all commentators have insisted that such a principle does govern the behavior of physicians.[5, 6]

Obviously, this principle cannot be interpreted as an ethical obligation on the physician to respond to any and every request for help; that would be physically impossible and financially ruinous for the practitioner. Thus, if there is such a principle, it must be limited in some way. The most obvious limits are choosing a specialty, selecting a geographical area, establishing a practice, and setting prices or a payment policy (which should include, if the overall principle is to be respected, some service at no or low fee). Other limits are clearly reprehensible, such as serving only the rich or persons of one race or religion. These limits make a mockery of the overall principle, as being rich or white or Catholic, for example, have nothing to do with medical need.

The most questionable limitation would be the exclusion of certain sorts of genuine, treatable medical needs because the physician finds something unacceptable about the need. For example, the disease renders the patient physically repugnant, the disease is associated with behavior the physician considers immoral, or—and this is the case with AIDS—the disease is dangerous to the physician. Clearly, refusing service for the first two reasons could not be justified, but is personal risk a reasonable excuse from service?

Historically, physicians regularly exposed themselves to serious risk when they treated the victims of infectious diseases. Physicians who fled from the scenes of epidemics have traditionally been criticized (though not always severely). Even when there is a presumption in favor of accepting risk in order to help those in need, the commonly accepted ethical rules for aiding others must be applied: Aid must be feasible, the risk must be reasonable, and there should be no less-risky alternatives.

The "reasonableness" of the risk in caring for patients with AIDS is the question. Reasonableness refers to such things as evidence that the activity is actually dangerous, the probability that evil will occur, and the magnitude of the evil for oneself and for others. Each of these elements must be assessed in light of the best available imformation and the best common sense about the situation at hand.

The best available information reveals that, in general, health workers are at very low risk of contracting HIV infection in performing the usual patient-care activities (see Chap. 14). The predominant studies confirm this, and of the cases of nosocomial HIV infection reported in the United States, most represent unusually intense exposure. At the same time, the best available information reveals that the magnitude of the evil is great: There is strong chance that infection will proceed to disease and that disease will lead to death.

Thus the moral quandary: Should I undertake an action that I have a presumed duty to perform if the action has a low probability of resulting in an evil for me (and others—for example, my spouse) of great magnitude? The best answer to that quandary, in the opinion of most commentators, is yes. The ethical rationale for that answer is that the duty to care for the sick is strong, and the avoidance of danger is a weak excuse to refuse to perform that duty unless the danger is imminent. Also, the implications of refusing needed care to certain "dangerous" patients are worrisome. Above all, a life ruled by the strategy of avoiding the low probabilities of even great harm would be a paralyzed life.

The answer would shift from a clear yes to a probably yes if the probability of harm increases or if the feasibility of helping decreases. Thus, doubt about the benefits of surgery or about its desirability to the patient, such as the proposal to place arterial access for hemodialysis in a terminally ill and demented AIDS patient, would strengthen the ethical justification of a refusal. Also, there may be imminent danger to unconsenting third parties, as when the surgeon may be pregnant. Thus, there are situations in which a physician or surgeon may make a plausible case that he or she will not treat a patient. However, it is obvious that psychological and emotional factors can heighten the sense of danger, magnify perceived risks, or reduce the apparent need or urgency of treatment. Scrupulous honesty and courage are indispensable adjuncts to such ethical evaluation.

A question less dramatic than actual refusal to treat is the proposal to require a preoperative test for HIV antibody of all surgical patients. Here the relevant question is what decisions might be faced and what procedures initiated on the basis of information gained by that test. Are there specific maneuvers that might be modified if the patient is antibody positive? For example, would the surgeon staple rather than suture, use a different technique for hemostasis, proceed more slowly and cautiously, pass instruments differently? If there are safer procedures that could be employed in the more dangerous (to the surgeon) situation, what increase in risk to the patient can be tolerated? Clearly, such reasoning can be part of a rational approach to care, and thus voluntary preoperative testing might be justified. At the same time, in the absence of any proposal about how the intervention could be managed more safely for the personnel and without detriment to the patient, there is a vivid possibility that information about the patient's seropositivity could lead to unjustified refusal of needed care. It goes without saying that such information, if disclosed, could be very prejudicial to the patient.

The conclusions, then, are that there is a strong imperative on physicians to respond to the need of the sick, that that imperative does allow certain limitations, but that a refusal to serve based on fear of disease is not easy to justify. It may be justified in certain situations, but only with sound reasons and honest reasoning.

Even when the reasoning points toward a justification, there are still matters that should give pause to anyone considering a refusal of a patient or contemplating a policy that would restrict the access of patients to needed care. The most compelling of these is, in my opinion, the importance of the work. AIDS is a significant health threat to this nation and to the world at this time. In the next decade, the numbers of patients and the magnitude of their need will grow, placing heavy burdens on the profession, on health care, and on the society. If members of the health professions exempt themselves from caring for these patients, they ignore the most serious task posed to their talents in this era. They would calmly contemplate from a distance the sight of thousands of sick and dying left unattended or attended only by those courageous professionals whose risks are now multiplied by their erstwhile colleagues who have retired to the sidelines. The refusal of one surgeon here and one nurse there may seem insignificant, but the occasional refusal, once tolerated, establishes a new principle in health care: Individuals may ethically ignore those in need of care. Such a principle fosters the perception that medicine is in no way different from a business, setting up shop where safe profits can be made.

This perception is a serious threat to the reputation of the profession and of all of its practitioners. Refusing treatment in specific cases casts a shadow on medicine's most precious value: its commitment to altruistic service. The words of a physician writing of the desertion of his colleagues during the Great London Plague of 1665 should be recalled: "Every man that undertakes to be of a profession or takes upon him any office must take all parts of it, the good and the evill, the pleasure and the pain, the profit and the inconvenience altogether and not pick and chuse, for ministers must preach, captains must fight, and physicians attend the sick."[7]

REFERENCES

1. AMA Council on Ethical and Judicial Affairs. *Current Opinions,* 1986, Principle VI, 9.11.
2. Zuger A, Miles SH. Physicians, AIDS, and occupational risk: Historical traditions and ethical obligations. *JAMA* 1987; 258:1924–1928.
3. *Code of Ethics of the America Medical Association,* 1847. Philadelphia: Turner Hamilton, 1871, p. 32.
4. AMA Council on Ethical and Judicial Affairs. Ethical issues involved in the growing AIDS crisis. *JAMA* 1988;259:1360–1361.
5. Arras JD. The fragile web of responsibility: AIDS and the duty to treat. *Hastings Center Report,* April 1988;10–20.
6. Walters L. Ethical issues in the prevention and treatment of HIV infection and AIDS. *Science* 1988;239:597–603.
7. Boghurst W. In: Payne, JF, ed. *Limographia*. London: 1894, p. 61.

16

AIDS: Educational and Research Resources

J. Brian O'Toole

The preceding chapters provide a summary of current knowledge about HIV infection and AIDS. An enormous amount of educational and research material is available to supplement the information presented in this book. The AIDS epidemic has prompted a multidisciplinary effort to further our understanding of this infection and to provide guidance for patient care.

In this chapter, a selected summary of available resources about HIV infection and AIDS is presented, including information about research programs, training efforts, organizations, and publications. Wherever possible, complete mailing addresses and telephone numbers are included; basic bibliographic retrieval information is provided for the publications listed.

INTERNATIONAL RESOURCES

AIDS Committee of Toronto
c/o Hassle Free Clinic
556 Church St., 2nd Floor
Toronto, Ontario, Canada K2P 1B6
416-922-0566 (women's telephone number)
416-922-0603 (men's telephone number)

AIDS Network of Edmonton
11303 102nd Ave.
Edmonton, Alberta, Canada T5K 0P6
403-426-1516

Collective d'Intervention Communautaire
Auprès des Gasis C.P. 29
O Succursal Victoria
Montréal, Québec, Canada
514-844-0010

Comité SIDA du Québec
3757 rue Prud'Homme
Montréal, Quebec, Canada H4A 3H8
514-282-9888

National Advisory Committee on AIDS
c/o Laboratory Centre for Disease Control
Health and Welfare Canada
Ottawa, Ontario, Canada K1A 0L2
613-990-8964

National AIDS Information Clearinghouse
P.O. Box 6003
Rockville, MD 20850
United States
301-762-5111 (reference assistance)
800-458-5231 (publications)
800-342-AIDS (hotline, English)
800-344-SIDA (hotline, Spanish)
800-AIDS-TTY (TDD/TTY, deaf and hard-of-hearing)

World Health Organization (WHO) AIDS Health Promotion Exchange
Special Program on AIDS
20 ave. Appi
1211 Geneva 27, Switzerland
Geneva: 001-4122-9121-11
WHO, New York office: 212-754-6000

NATIONAL RESOURCES

AIDS Action Committee
Health Care Provider Educator
661 Boylston St.
Boston, MA 02116
617-437-6250

AIDS Education Bureau
P.O. Box 272
Burke, VA 22015
703-323-5777

American Association of Blood Banks
1117 N. 19th St., Suite 600
Arlington, VA 22209
703-528-8200

American Association of Physicians for Human Rights
P.O. Box 14366
San Francisco, CA 94114
415-558-9353

American Dental Association
Richard Asa, Manager, Communications
211 E. Chicago Ave.
Chicago, IL 60611
312-440-2500

American Foundation for Aids Research (AmFAR)
40 W. 57th St., Suite 406
New York, NY 10019
212-333-3118

5900 Wilshire Blvd., 2nd Fl., East Satellite
Los Angeles, CA 90036
213-857-5900

AmFAR awards three types of grants:
Research grants of up to $50,000 for postdoctoral investigators;

Small grants (short-term travel grants) of up to $5,000 for short-term study or training at another U.S. institution; and

Scholar awards of up to $102,000 awarded over 3 years to investigators with 2–3 years of postdoctoral experience.

American Hospital Association
William H. Johnson, Jr., CEO
University of New Mexico Hospital
Chairman, Special Committee on AIDS/HIV Infections Policy
840 N. Lake Shore Drive
Chicago, IL 50511
312-280-6000

American Medical Association
AIDS Panel, Council on Scientific Affairs
535 N. Dearborn St.
Chicago, IL 60610
312-645-4430

American Medical Association AIDS Task Force
Robert Rinaldi, Ph.D., Task Force Contact
John J. Henning, Ph.D., AMA AIDS Coordinator
535 N. Dearborn St.
Chicago, IL 60611
312-280-5874

American Psychiatric Association AIDS Task Force
1400 K Street N.W.
Washington, DC
202-682-6000

American Red Cross National Headquarters, AIDS Education Office
1730 D St., N.W.
Washington, DC 20006
202-737-8300

American Osteopathic Association Task Force on AIDS
142 E. Ontario St.
Chicago, IL 60611
312-280-5874

American Public Health Association
William McBeath, M.D., Executive Director
1015 15th St., N.W.
Washington, DC 20005
202-789-5656

American Psychiatric Association AIDS Project
John Bonnage, Director
Stuart Nichols, M.D., Chairman
1400 K St., N.W.
Washington, DC 20005
202-682-6000

American Red Cross AIDS Education Office
1730 D St., N.W.
Washington, DC 20006
202-737-8300

Bureau of National Affairs, Inc.
1231 25th St., N.W.
Washington, DC 20039
800-452-7777; 202-452-4323

Centers for Disease Control Information and Education, Public Inquiries Office
1600 Clifton Rd., N.E.
Bldg. 1, Rm. B63
Atlanta, GA 30333
404-639-3311

Centers for Disease Control AIDS Information Office
1600 Clifton Rd. N.E.
Bldg. 6, Rm. 274
Atlanta, GA 30333
404-639-2891

Center for Interdisciplinary Research in Immunology and Disease
c/o Dept. of Microbiology and Immunology and Disease
UCLA School of Medicine
Los Angeles, CA 90024
213-825-1510

Coalition of Hispanic Health and Human Services Organizations
1030 15th St., N.W.
Washington, DC 20005
202-371-2100

Computerized AIDS Information Network
1213 N. Highland Ave.
Hollywood, CA 90038
213-464-7400 (ext. 277)

Department of Defense AIDS Program Activity: Health Information and Education
Program Specialist for Health Promotion
OASD (HA) PA&QA
Pentagon,
Washington, DC 20301
202-695-6800

Funders Concerned About AIDS
c/o Mrs. Joyce Bove, Chair
New York Community Trust
415 Madison Ave.
New York, NY 10017
212-758-0100
(Organization of grant makers interested in learning more about issues and sharing ideas about successful grants and techniques)

Intergovernmental Health Policy Project
2100 Pennsylvania Ave., N.W.
Washington, DC 20037
202-872-1455
(Maintains contact with states and legislative initiatives regarding AIDS; good resource documents)

Literature Search Program
Reference Section, National Library of Medicine
8600 Rockville Pike
Bethesda, MD 20894
(Note: starting in 1988, the National Library of Medicine publishes quarterly AIDS bibliography listings, which are available by subscription from the U.S. Government Printing Office for $12 a year. To order, request GPO List ID AID88 and send a check or money order to Superintendent of Documents, U.S. Government Printing Office, Washington, DC 20402, or telephone 202-783-3238)

National Academy of Sciences/Institute of Medicine
Theodore Cooper, Executive Vice President
The Upjohn Company, Chairman
AIDS Oversight Committee
National Academy of Sciences
2101 Constitution Ave., N.W.
Washington, DC 20418

National AIDS Information Clearinghouse
P.O. Box 6003
Rockville, MD 20850
301-762-5111 (reference assistance)
800-458-5231 (publications, bulk orders)
FAX: 301-738-6616
800-342-AIDS (hotline, English, publications, single copies)
800-344-SIDA (hotline, Spanish)
800-AIDS-TTY (TDD/TTY, deaf and hard-of-hearing)

In October 1987 the Centers for Disease Control, under the auspices of the U.S. Department of Health and Human Services, Public Health Service, established the National AIDS Information Clearinghouse (NAIC). The NAIC information network comprises the following components:

Resources Database: Information about more than 6000 governmental, educational, clinical, social services, religious, and other organizations that provide services and information related to AIDS and HIV infection. A subfile of this database is accessible via the National Library of Medicine's Directory of Information Resources Online.

Educational Materials Database: Information summarizing more than 2000 different types of educational materials, including videotapes, audiocassettes, posters, brochures, teaching guides, manuals, and additional formats. Some database information is included in the Combined Health Information Database, accessible via the Bibliographic Retrieval Service.

Reference Services: Staff provide information services through personal contact at meetings and via telephone requests regarding resources, programs, and services throughout the United States.

Publication Distribution Services: Distributes more than 60 free educational print materials; some materials are available in Spanish, Chinese, Portuguese, and braille.

Outreach Services: Provides health professionals with information on and contacts with various organizations, institutions, and agencies; provides a monthly calendar of upcoming events related to AIDS and HIV; provides a complete list of print materials available from the Clearinghouse and a NAIC *User Guide*.

National AIDS Network
2033 M St. N.W.
Suite 800
Washington, DC 20036
202-293-2437

National Cancer Institute's Physician Data Query
National Institutes of Health
Bldg. 82, Rm. 102
Bethesda, MD 20808
301-496-7403
(On-line computer system containing a directory of physicians and organizations that provide AIDS-related cancer care and file of active patient-treatment protocols)

National Center for Health Education
30 E. 29th St.
New York, NY 10016
212-689-1886

National Hemophilia Foundation, Metropolitan Chapter
104 E. 40th St.
New York, NY 10001
212-682-5510

National Hemophilia Foundation, National Headquarters
110 Greene St.
Rm. 406
New York, NY 10012
212-219-8180

P. O. Box 2644
Fairfax, VA 22031
703-352-2144

National Leadership Coalition on AIDS
1150 17th St., N.W.
Suite 202
Washington, D.C. 20036
202-429-0930

National Institute of Allergy and Infectious Diseases (NIAID)
A significant and functional resource for the physician in training, the AIDS treatment evaluation units are funded by NIAID at a number of medical schools throughout the country. The NIAID AIDS program is located at:

AIDS Treatment Evaluation Unit
Bldg. 31, No. 7-A48
Bethesda, MD 20892
301-496-5717.

A national toll-free telephone number is available for HIV-positive individuals who seek information on protocols, eligibility requirements, and the names of protocol directors: 800-TRIALS-A. Service is provided 9:00 A.M.–7:00 P.M. (EST), Monday–Friday.

National Institute of Drug Abuse–AIDS/Drug Abuse Information Clearinghouse
P.O. Box 2345
Rockville, MD 20852
301-468-2600

National Institutes of Health, Clinical Center
Bldg. 10, Rm. 1C-255
Bethesda, MD 20892
301-496-4891 (patient referral service);
Information on experimental drugs, 301-496-2563 or 301-496-5717

National Library of Medicine
4600 Rockville Pike
Bethesda, MD
301-496-4000

National Urban League
500 E. 62nd St.
New York, NY 10019
212-310-9000

Northwest AIDS Foundation
808 E. Pike
Seattle, WA 98122
206-329-6923

Physician's Association–AIDS Medical Resource Center
101 W. Grand Ave.
Rm. 200
Chicago, IL 60610
312-222-1326

Presidential Commission on the HIV Epidemic
655 15th St., N.W.
Suite 901
Washington, DC 20005
202-245-2437

Public Health Service National AIDS Hotline
800-342-AIDS (taped message and telephone number for specific questions; to speak with an operator call 800-342-7514)

Service Employees International Union AFL–CIO, CLC
1313 L St., N.W.
Washington, DC 20201

Robert Wood Johnson Foundation
P.O. Box 2316
Princeton, NJ 08543-2316
609-452-8701

The National Prison Project–AIDS Information
1616 P St., N.W.
Washington, DC 20036
202-331-0500

U.S. Public Health Service
Public Affairs Office
200 Independence Ave., S.W.
Hubert Humphrey Bldg., Rm. 725-H
Washington, DC 20201
202-245-6867

United Way of America
701 N. Fairfax St.
Alexandria, VA 22314-2045
703-836-7100

Veterans Administration
AIDS Education Task Force
VA Central Office
810 Vermont Ave., N.W.
Washington, DC 20420
202-223-3843

Workplace Health Communications Corporations
4 Madison Pl.
Albany, NY 12202

National Veterans Administration (VA) AIDS/HIV Training Coordinators

VA Regional Medical Education Center
Birmingham, AL
205-934-2105

VA Regional Medical Education Center
Long Beach, CA
213-494-5505

VA Medical Center
San Francisco, CA
415-221-4810

VA Central Office
Washington, DC
202-233-3843

VA Medical Center
Medical Education Center
Washington, DC
202-745-8301

VA Medical Center
Miami, FL
305-324-4455

VA Medical Center
Witchita, KS
316-685-2221

VA Regional Education Center
Minneapolis, MN
612-725-6537

VA Continuing Education Center
St. Louis, MO
314-894-6648

VA Medical Center
New York, NY
212-951-3346

VA Regional Medical Education Center
Northport, NY
516-261-4400

VA Regional Medical Education Center
Brecksville, OH
216-526-3030

VA Medical Center
Medical Education Center
Sioux Falls, SD
605-336-3230

VA Regional Medical Education Center
Salt Lake City, UT
801-582-1565

VA Medical Center
Martinsburg, VA
304-263-0811

VA Medical Center
Seattle, WA
206-762-1010

VA Medical Center
Madison, WI
608-262-7020

REGIONAL AND STATE RESOURCES

The Health Resources and Services Administration funds AIDS education and training centers, AIDS service demonstration projects, and pediatric AIDS health care demonstration projects nationwide. The Department of Health and Human Services and the Social Security Administration provide AIDS Coordinators in the 10 regions of the United States.

Health Resources and Services Administration

AIDS Education and Training Centers

CENTER	SERVICE AREA
New York University School of Education, Health, Nursing, and Arts Professions 429 Shimkin Hall Washington Square New York, NY 10003 212-998-5335	New York City and Long Island, New Jersey, Connecticut, Puerto Rico, Virgin Islands
University of Washington School of Medicine 820 N.E. 45th St., Suite 1 Seattle, WA 98105 206-543-9750	Washington, Oregon, Idaho, Alaska, Montana
Ohio State University Dept. of Family Medicine B0902 UHC, 456 W. 10th Ave. Columbus, OH 43210 614-293-8188	Ohio, Michigan, Kentucky, Tennessee
University of California, Davis Dept. of Family Practice California AHEC System Statewide Office 5110 E. Clinton Way Suite 115 Fresno, CA 93727-2098 209-252-2851	California, Nevada, Arizona, Hawaii
Emory University **School of Medicine** 735 Gatewood Road, N.E. Atlanta, GA 30322 404-727-2929	Alabama, Georgia, Florida, North Carolina, South Carolina
Louisiana State University Medical School 1542 Tulane Ave. New Orleans, LA 70112 504-568-3855	Arkansas, Louisiana, Mississippi

CENTER	SERVICE AREA
University of Colorado Health Science Center Colorado SEARCH/AHEC Program 4200 E. 9th Ave. Box A-096 Denver, CO 90262 303-270-5885	North Dakota, South Dakota, Utah, Colorado, New Mexico, Nebraska, Kansas, Wyoming
University of Illinois Dept. of Medical Social Work College of Associated Health Professions 808 S. Wood St. M/C 778, Rm. 173 Chicago, IL 60612 312-996-1373 and 312-996-1426	Iowa, Minnesota, Wisconsin, Illinois, Indiana, Missouri
University of Maryland at Baltimore Office of the Chancellor East Hall, 520 W. Lombard St. Baltimore, MD 21201 301-328-8334	Maryland, District of Columbia, Virginia, West Virginia, Delaware
University of Massachusetts Medical Center Massachusetts Statewide AHEC Program 55 Lake Ave. N. Worcester, MA 01655 617-856-3255	Maine, Massachusetts, New Hampshire, Rhode Island, Vermont
University of Southern California School of Medicine Dept. of Family Medicine 1420 San Pablo St. Los Angeles, CA 90033 213-224-7711	Five counties in Southern California (Los Angeles, Orange, Ventura, Riverside, San Bernadino)
University of Texas Health Science Center at Houston P.O. Box 20186 Houston, TX 77225 713-749-1011	Texas, Oklahoma
University of Pittsburg Reg. AIDS ETC, PA/NY Parran Hall, Rm. 207F Pittsburgh, PA 15261 412-624-1895	Pennsylvania, New York State (excluding New York City and Long Island)

Aids Service Demonstration Projects

Dept. of Health Services
1825 E. Roosevelt
Phoenix, AZ 85006
602-258-6381

Los Angeles County Dept. of Health Services
313 North Figueroa St.
Rm. 1014
Los Angeles, CA 90012
213-974-7803

Orange County Health Care Agency
515 North Sycamore
Santa Ana, CA 92701
714-834-2015

County of San Diego Dept. of Health Services
5454 Ruffin Rd.
Rm. 203
San Diego, CA 92133
619-495-5477

San Francisco Dept. of Public Health
1111 Market St.
3rd Fl.
San Francisco, CA 94103
415-864-5571

Dept. of Human Services Office of AIDS Activities
1660 L St., N.W.
Suite 700
Washington, DC 20036
202-673-3679

Public Health Trust of Dade County
Jackson Memorial Hospital
1611 N.W. 12th Ave.
Miami, FL 33136
305-549-7744

Comprehensive AIDS Program of Palm Beach County
3504 Broadway
West Palm Beach, FL 33407
407-845-4400

AIDS Atlanta
1132 W. Peachtree St.
Atlanta, GA 30309
404-872-0600

AIDS Foundation of Chicago
1332 N. Halsted St.
Chicago, IL 60622
312-642-5454

Associated Catholic Charities of New Orleans
New Orleans AIDS Project
1231 Prytania St.
New Orleans, LA 70130
504-523-3755

Fenway Community Health Center
93 Massachusetts Ave.
Boston, MA 02115
617-267-0900

New Jersey State Dept. of Health Div. of AIDS Prevention and Control, CN 363
363 W. State St.
Trenton, NJ 08625
609-984-6000

Health Research, Inc., and the New York State Dept. of Health
359 Corning Tower Bldg.
Albany, NY 12237
518-473-7238

Nassau-Suffolk Health System Agency
1537 Old Country Rd.
Planview, NY 11803
516-293-5740

Philadelphia Health Management Corp.
260 S. Broad St.
20th Fl.
Philadelphia, PA 19102-3890
215-985-2502

Community Council of Greater Dallas
AIDS ARMS Network
2121 Main St.
Suite 500
Dallas, TX 75201-4321
214-521-5191

Dept. of Health and Human Services
8000 N. Stadium Drive
Houston, TX 77054
713-794-9311

AIDS Health Service Program
1116 Summit Ave.
Suite 200
Seattle, WA 98101
206-587-4999

Puerto Rico Dept. of Health
Box 70184
San Juan, Puerto Rico 00936
809-766-1616

Pediatric AIDS Health Care Demonstration Projects

Case Management Demonstration Program, Los Angeles County
The Public Health Foundation of Los Angeles County
13200 Crossroads Parkway N.
Rm. 135
City of Industry, CA 91746
213-226-2406

Pediatric AIDS Health Care Demonstration Project
Public Health Trust–Dade County, Florida
1611 N.W. 12th Ave.
Miami, FL 33136
305-549-7744

Pediatric AIDS Demonstration Project
Georgia Dept. of Human Resources
Div. of Public Health
878 Peachtree St., N.E.
Rm. 217
Atlanta, GA 30309
404-894-6622

Pediatric AIDS Program
Children's Hospital of New Orleans
200 Henry Clay Ave.
New Orleans, LA 70118
504-899-9511

Boston Pediatric AIDS Project
Dimock Community Health Center
44 Dimock St.
Roxbury, MA 02119
617-442-8802

A Model Program for Pediatric AIDS Prevention and Control in Michigan
Michigan Dept. of Public Health
3423 N. Logan St.
P.O. Box 30195
Lansing, MI 48908
517-335-8368

New Jersey Dept. of Health Special Child Health Services, CN 364
Trenton, NJ 08625
609-292-5676

Family AIDS Case Management Program
Human Resources Administration
250 Church St.
Rm. 1416
New York, NY 10013
212-553-5151

Northern Manhattan Women and Children's HIV Demonstration Project
Trustees of Columbia University
600 W. 168 St.
New York, NY 10032
212-928-5103

FACTS–Family AIDS Center for Treatment and Support
75 Davis St.
Providence, RI 02908
401-277-2312

Pediatric AIDS Health Care Demonstration Project
University of Texas Health Science Center at San Antonio
7703 Floyd Curl Drive
San Antonio, TX 78284
512-567-5202

Seattle-King County Pediatric AIDS Demonstration Project
Seattle-King County Dept. of Public Health
110 Prefontaine Place South
Suite 500
Seattle, WA 98104
206-587-2797

Puerto Rico Pediatric AIDS Demonstration Project
Puerto Rico Dept. of Health
Box 70184
San Juan, Puerto Rico 00936
809-765-6210

Department of Health and Human Services and the Social Security Administration

Regional AIDS Coordinators

REGION	OFFICE
I	
Connecticut, Maine, Massachusetts, New Hampshire, Rhode Island, Vermont	P.O. Box 9227* Boston, MA 02114 617-565-2881
	John F. Kennedy Federal Bldg.† Government Center Boston, MA 02203 617-565-1442
II	
New York, New Jersey, Puerto Rico, Virgin Islands	26 Federal Plaza* New York, NY 10278 212-264-7291
	Jacob K. Javits Federal Bldg.† 26 Federal Plaza New York, NY 10278 212-264-2560

REGION	OFFICE
III	
Delaware, District of Columbia, Maryland, Pennsylvania, Virginia, West Virginia	P.O. Box 8788* Philadelphia, PA 19191 215-596-6979
	Rm. 10140, Mail Stop 14† P.O. Box 13716 3535 Market St. Philadelphia, PA 19104
IV	
Alabama, Florida, Georgia, Kentucky, Mississippi, North Carolina, South Carolina, Tennessee	P.O. Box 1684* Atlanta, GA 30301 404-331-2475
	Max R. Pesses† 101 Marietta Tower Atlanta, GA 30323 404-331-2093 and 404-331-2313
V	
Illinois, Indiana, Michigan, Minnesota, Ohio, Wisconsin	300 S. Wacker Drive* 27th Fl. Chicago, IL 60606 312-353-1733
	300 S. Wacker Dr.† Chicago, IL 60606 312-353-3652
VI	
Arkansas, Louisiana, New Mexico, Oklahoma, Texas	1200 Main Tower* Rm. 1540 Dallas, TX 75202 214-767-4281
	1200 Main Tower† Dallas, TX 75202 214-767-3916

REGION	OFFICE
VII	
Iowa, Kansas, Missouri, Nebraska	601 E. 12th St.* Rm. 436 Kansas City, MO 64106 816-374-7257 601 E. 12th St.† Kansas City, MO 64106 816-374-3300
VIII	
Colorado, Montana, North Dakota, South Dakota, Utah, Wyoming	1961 Stout* Rm. 737 Denver, CO 80294 303-844-3346 1961 Stout St.† Denver, CO 80294 303-844-6166
IX	
Arizona, California, Guam, Nevada	100 Van Ness Ave.* 24th Fl. San Francisco, CA 94102 415-556-7029 Federal Office Bldg.† 50 United Nations Plaza San Francisco, CA 94102 415-556-2595
X	
Alaska, Idaho, Oregon, Washington	2901 Third Ave.* Mail 301 Seattle, WA 98121 206-442-4256 The Third and Broad Bldg.† 2901 Third Ave. Seattle, WA 98121 206-442-0430 206-442-0502

*Funded by the Social Security Administration.

†Funded by the Department of Health and Human Resources.

INFORMATION RETRIEVAL

Databases

Acquired Immune Deficiency Syndrome. London: Bureau of Hygiene and Tropical Disease.

AIDS Knowledge Base from San Francisco General Hospital. Cohen P, Sande MA, Volberding P, eds. Boston: Massachusetts Medical Society.

Biological Abstracts. Philadelphia: BIOSIS.

Computerized AIDS Information Network. Los Angeles, CA: Los Angeles Community Services Center and the California Dept. of Health Services.

Comprehensive Core Medical Library. Latham, NY: Bibliographic Retrieval System.

Computer Retrieval of Information on Scientific Projects. Bethesda, MD: National Library of Medicine.

Health Planning and Administration. Chicago: American Hospital Association.

International Pharmaceutical Abstracts. Bethesda, MD: American Society of Hospital Pharmacists.

MEDLINE. Bethesda, MD: National Library of Medicine.

Pharmaceutical News Index. Louisville, KY: Data Courier, Inc.

National AIDS Information Clearinghouse. Resources and educational materials databases. Washington, DC: U.S. Dept. of Health and Human Services. 301-762-5111 (Refer to details under National Resources section.)

AIDS-specific publications

AIDS, a Quarterly Bibliography for All Fields of Periodical Literature. Madison, WI: Lincoln Associates, 1987–.

AIDS Alert. Atlanta: American Health Consultants, 1986–.

AIDS: An International Bimonthly Journal. London: Gower Academic Journals, 1987–.

AIDS and Human Retroviruses Research. New York: Mary Ann Liebert, Inc., 1986–.

AIDS Business. Norwalk, CT: International Resource Development, Inc., 1987–.

AIDS Center News. Los Angeles: World Hemophilia AIDS Center, 1987–.

AIDS Clinical Care. Waltham, MA: Massachusetts Medical Society, 1989–.

AIDS Clinical Digest. Atlanta: American Health Consultants, 1988–.

AIDS Crisis. Boca Raton, FL: Social Issues Resources Series, 1987–.

AIDS Educator. San Francisco, CA: San Francisco AIDS Foundation, 1987–.

AIDS Forum. Scottsdale, AZ: AIDS Forum, 1987–.

AIDS Health Promotion Exchange. Geneva: World Health Organization, Special Program on AIDS, 1988–.

AIDS Information Exchange. Washington, DC: U.S. Conference of Mayors, 1986–.

AIDS Institute Newsletter. Albany, NY: New York State Dept. of Health, 1985–.

AIDS Literature and News Review. Frederick, MD: University Publishers Group, 1987–.

AIDS Medical Update. Los Angeles: Center for Interdisciplinary Research in Immunology and Diseases at UCLA, 1983–.

AIDS Monthly Field Activities Report. Sacramento: Dept. of Health Services, 1986–.

AIDS Nursing Update. Los Angeles AIDS Clinical Research Center, 1987–.

AIDS Patient Care. New York: Mary Ann Liebert, Inc., 1987–.

AIDS Policy and Law. Washington, DC: Buraff Publications, 1986–.

AIDS Practice Manual, A Legal and Educational Guide. San Francisco: National Gay Rights Advocates and the National Lawyers' Guild, 1986–.

AIDS Prevention. Culpeper, VA: National AIDS Prevention Institute, 1987–.

AIDS Record. Washington, DC: Biodata Publishers, 1987–.

AIDS Research and Human Retroviruses. New York: Mary Ann Liebert, Inc., 1985–.

AIDS Research Today. Philadelphia: BIOSIS, 1987–.

AIDS Research. New York: Mary Ann Liebert, Inc., 1983–1985.

AIDS Targeted Information Newsletter. Baltimore: Williams & Wilkins, 1987–.

AIDS Update. New York: Lambda Legal Defense and Education Fund, Inc., 1987–.

AIDS Update. Los Angeles, CA: Center for Health Resources, 1987–.

AIDS Update. New York: National Gay Task Force, 1985–.

AIDS Update Newsletter. Saratoga, CA: R&E Publishers, 1986–.

AIDSFILE. San Francisco: San Francisco General Hospital, 1986–.

Archives of AIDS Research. Kiawah Island, SC: Reproductive Health Center, 1987–.

Bulletin of Experimental Treatments for AIDS. San Francisco: San Francisco AIDS Foundation, 1987–.

California AIDS Update. Sacramento: Senator David Roberti, 1985–.

CDC AIDS Weekly. Atlanta: Charles Hamilton, 1986–.

Current AIDS Literature. London: Gower Academic Journals, 1988–.

DAIR Update. San Francisco: Documentation of AIDS Issues and Research, Inc., 1986–.

Focus: A Guide to AIDS Research. San Francisco: San Francisco AIDS Health Project, 1985–.

Hemophilia Information Exchange. New York: National Hemophilia Foundation, 1986–.

Journal of the Acquired Immune Deficiency Syndrome. New York: Raven Press, 1988–.

NAN Multi-Cultural Notes. Washington, DC: National AIDS Network, 1986–.

NAN Monitor. Washington, DC: National AIDS Network, 1986–.

Network News. Washington, DC: National AIDS Network, 1986–.

Quarterly Report to the Legislature on HTLV-III Antibody Alternative Test Site Program. Sacramento: Dept. of Health Services, Preventive Health Services, 1985–.

PAAC Notes. Chicago: Physicians' Association for AIDS.

San Francisco AIDS Foundation News. San Francisco, 1985–.

State AIDS Reports. Washington, DC: Intergovernmental Health Policy Project, 1988–.

REFERENCES

AIDS Resource Listing, Selected CDC Guidance. Bethesda, MD: U.S. Dept. of Health and Human Services, 1989.

AIDS Resources Listing, Information Contacts. Bethesda, MD: U.S. Dept. of Health and Human Services, 1989.

Flaskerud, JH, ed. AIDS/HIV Infection, *A Reference Guide for Nursing Professionals*. Philadelphia: W. B. Saunders, 1989.

Frontline Healthcare, AIDS Education and Training. Bethesda, MD: Workplace Resources, 1989.

Halleron TA, Disaneschi JI, eds., *AIDS Infection Resources Directory*. Washington, DC, 1988.

Lindsay T, et al. *AIDS, A Guide to Research Resources*. Berkeley, CA: The Library, University of California at Berkeley, 1988.

17

AIDS Continuing Medical Education Self-Assessment

Paul G. Ramsey

The following questions have been developed from the material presented in this handbook for the purpose of allowing you to assess your understanding and retention of the material presented and to receive continuing medical education (CME) credit.

The University of Washington School of Medicine designates this CME activity for 9 credit hours in Category 1 of the Physician's Recognition Award of the American Medical Association, provided that it is used and completed as directed.

To receive a transcript verifying the credit earned, the reader should first review the material contained in the handbook and respond to the items contained in the self-assessment examination. Mark your answers by circling the letter corresponding to your choice of the correct answer on the answer sheet at the end of the examination. The completed answer sheet, the application for credit, and the handbook evaluation form should be mailed with a check or money order for $20 to:

AIDS Handbook Section, Continuing Medical Education
University of Washington School of Medicine
1325 Fourth Avenue, Suite 2000
Seattle, WA 98101

Credit will be awarded only to those individuals who attain a score of 60% or higher. An analysis of the examination items with an explanation will be sent to all who submit the application for credit. This self-assessment examination must be submitted for credit purposes before July 30, 1991.

In accordance with the ACCME, the self-assessment examination and this book have been planned, developed, and produced by members of the faculty of the University of Washington in cooperation with McGraw-Hill Publishing Company.

AIDS CME SELF-ASSESSMENT

1. All of the following may be characteristic of patients classified by CDC criteria as having Group I HIV infection **except**:
   a. Patients may have aseptic meningitis
   b. Symptoms may resemble those of mononucleosis, with malaise, fever, lymphadenopathy, rash, and headache
   c. Symptoms usually occur 1–12 weeks after acute exposure to HIV
   d. Patients may have persistent lymphadenopathy for more than 4 months
   e. Symptoms are usually self-limited

2. Based on the CDC classification system, which class of patients would invariably be asymptomatic?
   a. Group I
   b. Group II
   c. Group III
   d. Group IV

3. The key finding that places patients with HIV infection in CDC Group III is the following:
   a. Significant weight loss
   b. Persistent lymphadenopathy (greater than 1 cm in diameter) for at least 3 months
   c. Opportunistic infections
   d. An asymptomatic status
   e. Laboratory abnormalities such as leukopenia, lymphopenia, thrombocytopenia, hypergammaglobulinemia, or anemia

4. All of the following conditions characterize patients who would be classified by CDC criteria as Group IV **except**:
   a. Neurologic disease
   b. Symptoms previously defined as ARC
   c. Persistent diarrhea or weight loss
   d. Constitutional symptoms and wasting
   e. Usually an asymptomatic status

5. Which of the following is the most common opportunistic infection in patients with HIV infection?
   a. Oral candidiasis
   b. *Pneumocystis carinii* pneumonia (PCP)

c. CMV infection
d. Tuberculosis
e. *Salmonella* bacteremia

6. All of the following cause esophagitis in patients with HIV infection **except**:
   a. *Candida albicans*
   b. Herpes simplex virus
   c. CMV
   d. *Pneumocystis carinii*

7. Which of the following is **not** currently used for diagnosing PCP?
   a. Examination of induced sputum
   b. Examination of fluid from nasotracheal suction
   c. Serologic tests
   d. Examination of transbronchial biopsy material
   e. Examination of fluid from bronchoalveolar lavage

8. Current evidence suggests that chemoprophylaxis for PCP in patients with AIDS is indicated for persons who have recovered from an episode of PCP or patients with Kaposi's sarcoma undergoing chemotherapy. All of the following appear to be useful chemoprophylactic regimens **except**:
   a. Trimethoprim-sulfamethoxazole, one double-strength tablet twice daily
   b. Zidovudine, 100 mg six times daily
   c. Dapsone, 100 mg daily
   d. Inhaled pentamidine, twice a month

9. Which of the following is the most useful diagnostic test for *Mycobacterium avium intracellulare* infection in persons with AIDS?
   a. Skin test
   b. Blood cultures
   c. Cultures of expectorated sputum
   d. Skin biopsy
   e. Serologic tests

10. Which of the following opportunistic viral infections commonly associated with HIV infection causes the most devastating visual problems?
    a. Herpes simplex virus
    b. CMV
    c. Adenovirus
    d. Influenza virus
    e. Coxsackievirus

11. The following descriptions characterize Kaposi's sarcoma **except**:
   a. Patients frequently do not have cutaneous involvement
   b. Gastrointestinal involvement, including the mouth, is common
   c. Lesions may be erythematous, purple, or multicolored
   d. Yellow halos around lesions are common
   e. Early lesions may be difficult to distinguish from bruises

12. The most common presentation of HIV infection as a neurologic syndrome is:
   a. Meningitis
   b. Focal neurologic signs with mass lesions found by CT scans
   c. Spinal cord syndromes
   d. Asymmetric peripheral neuropathy
   e. AIDS dementia complex

13. The most common cause of central nervous system mass lesions in patients with HIV infection is:
   a. *Mycobacterium tuberculosis*
   b. CMV
   c. *Cryptococcus neoformans*
   d. *Toxoplasma gondii*
   e. Lymphoma

14. A patient with AIDS who has had multiple opportunistic infections in the past presents with focal neurologic signs. A CT scan of the head shows a mass lesion in an area of the brain that would be difficult for the neurosurgeon to biopsy. A reasonable approach to this patient's problem would be:
   a. Empiric therapy with sulfadiazine and pyrimethamine
   b. Empiric therapy with amphotericin B
   c. Empiric therapy with antituberculous medications
   d. Consultation with an oncologist about chemotherapy for lymphoma
   e. Encourage the neurosurgeon to obtain a biopsy specimen

15. The most common cause of meningitis in patients with HIV infection is:
   a. *Toxoplasma gondii*
   b. *Cryptococcus neoformans*
   c. *Mycobacterium tuberculosis*
   d. Herpes simplex virus
   e. CMV

16. The most frequent acute organic mental disorder seen in patients with AIDS is:
   a. Manic depression

b. Schizophrenia
c. Delirium
d. Violent behavior

17. All of the following should lead to suspicion of early dementia in patients with AIDS **except**:
a. Hypersomnia
b. Impaired judgment
c. Handwriting changes
d. Increased sensitivity to alcohol
e. Increased fatigue

18. Which of the following would be a reasonable medication regimen to begin treating a patient with AIDS for depression?
a. High-dose tricyclic antidepressants
b. Lower than usual doses of tricyclic antidepressants
c. Monoamine oxidase inhibitors
d. Benzodiazepines
e. Lithium

19. All of the following statements correctly characterize the risk of transmission of HIV from an infected patient to a health care worker **except**:
a. There is an approximately 0.4 percent risk of seroconversion for hospital employees after needlestick or other sharp injury exposure to the blood of HIV-infected patients
b. The risk of transmission of HIV is approximately the same as the risk of transmission of hepatitis B virus
c. The risk of HIV infection is extremely low after a health care worker is exposed to blood that does not involve penetrating injuries
d. A negative HIV antibody test 3 months after a needlestick injury does not rule out all possibility of HIV infection

20. All of the following statements correctly characterize the body substance isolation policy for prevention of the spread of HIV infection **except**:
a. Health care workers should wear gloves when contacting any patient's blood
b. Patients with AIDS do not routinely need private rooms
c. Needles should be capped immediately after blood is drawn
d. Gloves should be worn for examination of all patients' mouths
e. Laboratory specimens from all patients should be handled in the same manner

21. Which of the following is an effective infection control practice?
a. Masks worn when examining patients with AIDS
b. Use of disposable plates and eating utensils
c. Protective isolation of patients with AIDS
d. Use of gloves when contacting mucous membranes of all patients
e. Wearing gowns for examining all patients

22. The most common risk factor leading to HIV infection in women in the United States is:
a. Blood transfusions
b. Homosexual contacts
c. IV drug use by self or sexual partner
d. Prostitution

23. All of the following statements characterize a reasonable policy for antepartum screening of pregnant women for HIV infection **except**:
a. A policy based on screening for known risk factors for HIV infection would detect more than 90 percent of HIV-infected women
b. In the United States, all pregnant women should be offered HIV screening as part of their prenatal care with appropriate pre- and posttest counseling
c. Seronegative women who engage in high-risk behaviors should receive appropriate education regarding risk reduction and should be rescreened during the third trimester
d. A woman's potential response to a positive HIV test should be assessed during pretest counseling

24. All of the following statements correctly characterize the approach to intrapartum care for HIV-seropositive and -seronegative pregnant women **except**:
a. Universal body substance isolation procedures should be maintained during delivery for all patients
b. Parenteral therapy (such as vitamin K or heelstick hematocrits) for the infant should be delayed until after stabilization and bathing to avoid inoculating HIV through the skin during all deliveries
c. Mode of delivery is determined by usual obstetric indications
d. Known HIV infection is an indication for cesarean section
e. Procedures such as fetal scalp electrode placement and fetal blood sampling that potentially increase the exposure of fetal blood to maternal secretions should be avoided when possible

25. Most pediatric cases of AIDS are related to:
a. Treatment for hemophilia
b. Exposure to contaminated blood products

c. Perinatal acquisition of infection
d. Postnatal transmission from infected parent

26. Which of the following is a correct statement about the diagnosis of HIV infection in a 12-month-old baby?
a. Traditional antibody testing techniques (ELISA and Western blot) are adequate to diagnose an infected 12-month-old baby
b. Laboratory identification of HIV-infected 12-month-old babies requires direct detection of virus or viral antigen
c. Development of new HIV bands on sequential Western blot tests does not indicate HIV infection
d. Twelve-month-old babies who are infected with HIV can always be diagnosed by symptoms and signs of HIV infection

27. All of the following are more frequent manifestations of AIDS in children than in adults **except**:
a. Lymphoid interstitial pneumonitis
b. Bacterial meningitis
c. PCP
d. Bacterial pneumonia
e. Bacteremia

28. Children in the United States with symptomatic HIV infection should receive all of the following immunizations **except**:
a. *Hemophilus influenzae* type B conjugate vaccine
b. Pneumococcal vaccine
c. Influenza virus vaccine
d. Oral polio vaccine
e. Measles, mumps, and rubella vaccine

29. The most common opportunistic disease found in children with AIDS is:
a. Disseminated CMV infection
b. *Candida* esophagitis
c. Lymphoid interstitial pneumonitis
d. Herpes simplex virus infection
e. PCP

30. Recognized causes of diarrhea in HIV-infected patients include all of the following **except**:
a. *Shigella* species
b. *Cryptosporidium* species
c. *Isospora belli*
d. *Mycobacterium* species
e. All of the above

31. Antimicrobial therapy appears to be effective for treating all of the following organisms **except**:
a. *Isospora belli*
b. *Campylobacter* species
c. *Cryptosporidium* species
d. *Shigella* species

32. Antimicrobial therapy is effective for treating pulmonary infection with all of the following organisms **except**:
a. *Mycobacterium avium intracellularae*
b. *Pneumocystis carinii*
c. *Mycobacterium tuberculosis*
d. *Cyptococcus neoformans*
e. Gram-negative bacteria

33. A characteristic feature that helps to distinguish oral candidiasis from hairy leukoplakia is:
a. Absence of associated opportunistic infections
b. Presence of white plaques
c. Presence of dysphagia
d. Cough
e. Oral lesions nonadherent to the mucosal surface

34. All of the following infectious agents have been reported to cause cutaneous disease in patients with HIV infection **except**:
a. *Entamoeba histolytica*
b. *Candida albicans*
c. *Cryptococcus neoformans*
d. *Cryptosporidium* species
e. *Histoplasma capsulatum*

35. Which of the following skin conditions are associated with AIDS?
a. Urticaria
b. Severe seborrhea
c. Generalized erythroderma
d. Severe psoriasis
e. All of the above

36. All of the following statements correctly describe psychosocial issues related to the diagnosis of ARC **except**:
a. Patients with ARC may undergo depression
b. Patients with ARC are keenly interested in their doctors' opinions of ways to prevent progression to AIDS

c. Patients with ARC experience lower levels of emotional distress than patients with full-blown AIDS
d. Patients with ARC are at risk for developing neuropsychiatric problems such as cognitive dysfunction

37. All of the following are correct statements about the care of an asymptomatic individual who is seropositive for HIV infection **except**:
a. An initial biomedical evaluation should be performed to determine whether a patient truly lacks symptoms or signs and to gather baseline information
b. Ongoing screening for disease progression and opportunistic infections should be planned
c. No prophylactic measures are indicated initially
d. Education concerning prevention of HIV transmission is important
e. Identification and strengthening of psychological and social supports are important components of care

38. Which of the following components of the physical examination should be repeated frequently (e.g., at least every 6 months) in patients who are asymptomatic but HIV seropositive?
a. Fundoscopic examination
b. Examination for lymphadenopathy
c. Oral examination
d. Detailed skin examination
e. All of the above

39. All of the following are true statements about beta-2 microglobulin **except**:
a. Beta-2 microglobulin is a protein that is part of the major histocompatibility complex
b. Serum levels of beta-2 microglobulin are thought to reflect lymphocyte turnover
c. Cohort studies show that increased levels of beta-2 microglobulin correlate with increased risk of progressing to AIDS
d. Increased levels of beta-2 microblobulin do not correlate with increased risk of progressing to AIDS independent of CD4 lymphocyte counts
e. Beta-2 microglobulin is used in other settings for evaluation of immune function and is generally available

40. An otherwise asymptomatic, HIV-seropositive patient presents with new onset of cough, rhinitis, and mild general malaise for the past 2 days. The patient had recent T-lymphocyte studies that showed that his CD4 cell count was 800. There are no abnormalities on physical examination, and the patient is afebrile, with a normal respiratory rate. Which of the following approaches would you use for this patient?

a. Gallium scan
b. Chest x-ray
c. Arterial blood gas measurement
d. Hospitalization
e. Careful follow-up of the patient without initial tests

41. Which of the following screening tests should **not** be performed in an asymptomtic patient who is HIV seropositive?

a. VDRL
b. CBC
c. CD4:CD8 ratio determination
d. Tuberculin skin test (PPD)
e. Stool examination for ova and parasites

42. Which of the following statements best characterizes the role of zidovudine for an asymptomatic patient who is seropositive for HIV?

a. Evidence suggests that there is no role for zidovudine for the asymptomatic patient
b. Zidovudine should be used for all asymptomatic patients because the benefits clearly outweigh the risks
c. Accumulating evidence suggests that zidovudine may be effective as a prophylactic agent when started for asymptomatic patients with HIV infection who have CD4 cell counts less than 500
d. Zidovudine should be offered to partners of asymptomatic patients who are seropositive for HIV

43. All of the following are true statements about tuberculosis in patients with HIV infection **except**:

a. The CDC has found that patients with AIDS with active *Mycobacterium tuberculosis* infection respond well to conventional antituberculous treatment
b. HIV-seropositive, asymptomatic patients should receive tuberculin skin testing and chemoprophylaxis if they are found to be reactive
c. An attack rate of nearly 8 percent per year among HIV-infected patients has been reported
d. Current data show that there is no need to give isoniazid chemoprophylaxis for more than 1 year for HIV-infected patients who are PPD positive
e. CD4 cell counts are used by some physicians to guide decisions about whether to continue isoniazid prophylaxis for more than 1 year

44. All of the following are recommended **as part of an annual examination** for asymptomatic, HIV-seropositive patients who are not anergic **except**:
a. T-lymphocyte studies
b. CBC
c. Chest x-ray
d. VDRL
e. Tuberculin skin test (PPD) with anergy battery

45. The mechanism of action of zidovudine against HIV appears to be:
a. Interruption of HIV binding to target cells
b. Interference with viral budding
c. Inhibition of reverse transcriptase, preventing transcription of RNA to DNA
d. Interference with DNA integration into the host genome
e. Inhibition of viral component production and assembly

46. Clinical trials with zidovudine suggest all of the following **except**:
a. A decrease in mortality due to opportunistic infections in patients with AIDS or ARC treated with zidovudine compared with patients treated with placebo
b. Improved neuropsychiatric function in patients treated with zidovudine compared to patients treated with placebo
c. Reduction in circulating levels of HIV core protein in zidovudine-treated patients compared to placebo-treated patients
d. Absence of serious side effects in zidovudine-treated patients with AIDS or ARC
e. Increased blood transfusion requirements in patients treated with zidovudine compared to those treated with placebo

47. Reported side effects of zidovudine include all of the following **except**:
a. Anemia
b. Neutropenia
c. Nausea
d. Confusion
e. Increased opportunistic infections

48. A patient with early ARC with a CD4 cell count of 300/mm^3 was started on zidovudine at a dose of 200 mg five times a day 3 months ago. He now complains of fatigue and dizziness upon sitting up. The patient shows an increase in pulse rate by 25 beats per minute standing and a decrease in blood pressure by 15 mm Hg. His hematocrit is 30 mg%, decreased from 39 mg%. The mean corpuscular volume is 106, the mean corpuscular hemoglobin is 32. Total neutrophils are 850. Appropriate actions include all the following **except**:

a. A reduction in zidovudine to 100 mg five times daily.
b. Determination of the serum erythropoietin level.
c. Determination of the serum folate level.
d. Granulocyte transfusion.

49. Currently zidovudine is approved by the FDA for the following indications:

a. Patients with overt AIDS or patients with symptomatic ARC with fewer than 200 circulating CD4 cells
b. Asymptomatic, HIV-seropositive patients with CD4 cell counts below 500
c. Asymptomatic patients with ARC with fewer than 200 circulating CD4 cells
d. All of the above

50. Which of the following statements describes the position of the AMA and other medical organizations about a physician's duty to treat patients with AIDS?

a. Neither patients who have AIDS nor those who have been infected with HIV should be subject to discrimination based on fear or prejudice
b. A physician may ethically refuse to treat any patient whose condition is within the physician's realm of competence
c. The best available information suggests that health care workers are at such high risk of contracting HIV infection in providing the usual patient care activities that physicians can ethically refuse to perform nonelective procedures
d. All of the above

51. Appropriate reasons for a physician to recommend HIV antibody testing for a patient include all of the following **except**:

a. Signs suggestive of HIV infection, such as hairy leukoplakia
b. Persistent, unexplained symptoms for more than 2 weeks, such as diarrhea, night sweats, or lymphadenopathy
c. Identification of an unexplained opportunistic pathogen
d. Excessive concern about AIDS in patients with no identified risk factors
e. Patients with a significant risk for acquisition of HIV

52. For men, all of the following constitute probable risk factors for acquiring HIV infection **except**:

a. Unprotected anal or oral intercourse with other men prior to 1975

b. Multiple blood transfusions received after 1975 and before 1985
c. Unprotected anal or oral intercourse with other men after 1975
d. Hemophilia and treatment with multiple blood products after 1975 and before 1985
e. Multiple sexual contacts with prostitutes

53. A potential contraindication to recommending an immediate HIV antibody test for a patient is:
a. A history of previous positive VDRL
b. A history of recent opportunistic infection
c. An asymptomatic patient with a normal CBC
d. A depressed patient who appears to be suicidal
e. A patient with risk factors for HIV infection who will be moving to another state in the near future

54. All of the following are true statements about the ELISA HIV antibody test **except**:
a. The positive predictive value of the ELISA (the likelihood that a positive ELISA actually represents true HIV infection) is dependent on the prior probability of HIV infection in an individual (presence of risk factors)
b. The strength of ELISA reactivity (strongly versus borderline reactive) affects the predictive value of the test
c. For individuals with no known risk of HIV infection, the probability that a positive ELISA reflects true HIV infection is approximately 20 percent
d. The HIV ELISA test is highly sensitive (at least 99 percent) and highly specific (99 percent)
e. Most laboratories will report positive ELISA results without confirmatory test results

55. All of the following are true statements about the Western blot test **except**:
a. Indeterminate Western blot results can be reported in both low- and high-risk persons in as many as 25 percent of ELISA-reactive specimens
b. False-negative Western blot tests never occur in individuals at high risk for HIV infection
c. False-positive Western blot tests are almost never found in persons who are at high risk for HIV infection
d. The Western blot test detects antibodies to specific viral antigens
e. The Western blot test is time-consuming and subjective, with some interlaboratory variability in technique and interpretation

56. All of the following statements are true about HIV antibody tests **except**:

a. Indeterminate HIV Western blots are due to early seroconversion, autoantibodies, and possible cross-reactivity with antibodies to other viruses

b. A confirmatory test is not necessary if the HIV ELISA is positive

c. A low-risk individual with an indeterminate Western blot should be followed for 6 months with repeat Western blots and should be counseled that he or she is unlikely to be infected with HIV if a Western blot is negative or indeterminate after 6 months of follow-up

d. False-negative antibody tests have been reported in high-risk individuals with evidence of HIV infection by culture in 3 years of follow-up

e. The likelihood (i.e., positive predictive value) that an individual is infected with HIV as determined by a reactive ELISA followed by a positive Western blot is 99 percent in high-risk individuals and 93–99 percent in low-risk individuals

57. During pretest counseling concerning the HIV antibody test, it is important to include all of the following **except**:

a. Education about the modes of HIV transmission and methods of reducing risk of transmission

b. The nature, purpose, and consequences of HIV testing

c. Assessment of the patient's risk of infection with HIV

d. Assessment of the patient's ability to cope with the result if the test is positive

e. Discussion of the advantages of early treatment with zidovudine if the HIV test is positive

58. In taking a history from a new male patient concerning the possible risk of HIV infection, a clinician should:

a. Ask open-ended questions in a nonjudgmental fashion

b. Ask about previous STDs

c. Ask questions in the appropriate vernacular about drug use

d. Ask "have you had sex with men, or women, or both?"

e. All of the above

59. In providing counseling after an HIV test has been performed, a clinician should do all of the following **except**:

a. Meet in person with patients who are at risk for HIV infection

b. Delay presenting the result of the HIV test until the end of the counseling session, when the patient fully understands the implications

c. Interpret the meaning of a positive or indeterminate result
d. Discuss plans for medical or psychological services for newly diagnosed, HIV-seropositive patients
e. Discuss the importance of safer sex and drug practices

60. Human retroviruses are divided into two subfamilies, the transforming oncoviruses and the cytopathic lentiviruses, which share which of the following characteristics:
a. Lack of budding from the cell surface
b. Absence of an envelope
c. A high molecular weight, single-stranded DNA genome
d. Encoding of an RNA-dependent DNA polymerase (reverse transcriptase)
e. All of the above

61. HTLV-I or HTLV-II may do the following **except**:
a. Cause adult T-cell leukemia
b. Lead to degenerative central nervous system disease
c. Cause tropical spastic paraparesis
d. Cause hairy cell leukemia
e. Cause AIDS

62. True statements about lentiviruses include all of the following **except**:
a. Lentiviruses are morphologically distinct from HTLV-I and HTLV-II
b. Two types of human lentiviruses have been fully characterized (HIV-1 and HIV-2)
c. Lentiviruses cause slowly progressive disease with lymphotropic and neurotropic features
d. Lentiviruses cause disease exclusively in humans
e. Lentiviruses produce cytopathology in their target cells, including syncytium formation

63. Which of the following best describes the usual pattern of in vivo viral expression associated with HIV?
a. Latent infection characterized by intermittent episodes of acute disease, with no virus detected between episodes
b. Chronic active infection in which infectious virus is always demonstrable although disease may be absent
c. Persistent infection characterized by a long incubation period with slowly increasing amounts of virus
d. All of the above

64. An important property of HIV that may lead to development of resistance to some potential chemotherapeutic agents is:

a. Autoimmune destruction of CD4 cells
b. Hypervariability in the HIV *env* gene
c. Ability of HIV to infect and kill the CD4 lymphocyte
d. Antigenic stimulation and subsequent differentiation of an HIV-infected CD4 cell

65. Which of the following have been documented as modes of transmission of HIV?
a. Bites by mosquitos or other arthropods
b. Contamination of mucous membranes with saliva
c. Sharing eating utensils
d. All of the above
e. None of the above

66. Which of the following has (have) been implicated as cofactor(s) that enhance the efficiency of sexual transmission of HIV?
a. Genital ulcer disease
b. Intact foreskin (i.e., absence of circumcision)
c. Advanced immunodeficiency in the infected person
d. All of the above
e. None of the above

67. Which of the following most accurately represents the relative efficiencies of HIV transmission?
a. Transfusion > receptive intercourse > insertive intercourse
b. Receptive intercourse > transfusion > insertive intercourse
c. Transfusion > insertive intercourse > receptive intercourse
d. Receptive intercourse > insertive intercourse > transfusion
d. Insertive intercourse > receptive intercourse > transfusion

68. Which of the following most accurately summarizes trends in heterosexually acquired AIDS in the United States from 1981 to 1989?
a. Percentage of cases in patients born outside the United States **increasing,** percentage with domestic heterosexual exposure **declining**
b. Percentage of cases in patients born outside the United States **declining,** percentage with domestic heterosexual exposure **increasing**
c. Percentage of cases in patients born outside the United States and percentage with domestic heterosexual exposure **both increasing**
d. Percentage of cases in patients born outside the United States and percentage with domestic heterosexual exposure **both declining**
d. None of the above

AIDS CME SELF-ASSESSMENT ANSWER SHEET

Please circle your response to each of the 68 questions in the self-assessment examination; check the number of each question as you mark the answer to ensure that you are responding to the intended question.

1. (a)(b)(c)(d)(e)
2. (a)(b)(c)(d)(e)
3. (a)(b)(c)(d)(e)
4. (a)(b)(c)(d)(e)
5. (a)(b)(c)(d)(e)
6. (a)(b)(c)(d)(e)
7. (a)(b)(c)(d)(e)
8. (a)(b)(c)(d)(e)
9. (a)(b)(c)(d)(e)
10. (a)(b)(c)(d)(e)
11. (a)(b)(c)(d)(e)
12. (a)(b)(c)(d)(e)
13. (a)(b)(c)(d)(e)
14. (a)(b)(c)(d)(e)
15. (a)(b)(c)(d)(e)
16. (a)(b)(c)(d)(e)
17. (a)(b)(c)(d)(e)
18. (a)(b)(c)(d)(e)
19. (a)(b)(c)(d)(e)
20. (a)(b)(c)(d)(e)
21. (a)(b)(c)(d)(e)
22. (a)(b)(c)(d)(e)
23. (a)(b)(c)(d)(e)
24. (a)(b)(c)(d)(e)
25. (a)(b)(c)(d)(e)
26. (a)(b)(c)(d)(e)
27. (a)(b)(c)(d)(e)
28. (a)(b)(c)(d)(e)
29. (a)(b)(c)(d)(e)
30. (a)(b)(c)(d)(e)
31. (a)(b)(c)(d)(e)
32. (a)(b)(c)(d)(e)
33. (a)(b)(c)(d)(e)
34. (a)(b)(c)(d)(e)
35. (a)(b)(c)(d)(e)
36. (a)(b)(c)(d)(e)
37. (a)(b)(c)(d)(e)
38. (a)(b)(c)(d)(e)
39. (a)(b)(c)(d)(e)
40. (a)(b)(c)(d)(e)
41. (a)(b)(c)(d)(e)
42. (a)(b)(c)(d)(e)
43. (a)(b)(c)(d)(e)
44. (a)(b)(c)(d)(e)
45. (a)(b)(c)(d)(e)
46. (a)(b)(c)(d)(e)
47. (a)(b)(c)(d)(e)
48. (a)(b)(c)(d)(e)
49. (a)(b)(c)(d)(e)
50. (a)(b)(c)(d)(e)
51. (a)(b)(c)(d)(e)
52. (a)(b)(c)(d)(e)
53. (a)(b)(c)(d)(e)
54. (a)(b)(c)(d)(e)
55. (a)(b)(c)(d)(e)
56. (a)(b)(c)(d)(e)
57. (a)(b)(c)(d)(e)
58. (a)(b)(c)(d)(e)
59. (a)(b)(c)(d)(e)
60. (a)(b)(c)(d)(e)
61. (a)(b)(c)(d)(e)
62. (a)(b)(c)(d)(e)
63. (a)(b)(c)(d)(e)
64. (a)(b)(c)(d)(e)
65. (a)(b)(c)(d)(e)
66. (a)(b)(c)(d)(e)
67. (a)(b)(c)(d)(e)
68. (a)(b)(c)(d)(e)

Please type or print.

____

Last name First name Middle initial

____

Address

____

City State Zip code

____

Social security number Specialty Degree Year of graduation

Please allow 4 weeks for processing.

AIDS Dx/Rx EVALUATION

Please complete the following evaluation by circling the number that best represents your response to the question.

1. The handbook improved my knowledge about AIDS.	Strongly agree			Strongly disagree	
	(1)	(2)	(3)	(4)	(5)
2. The handbook has a good educational format.	Strongly agree			Strongly disagree	
	(1)	(2)	(3)	(4)	(5)
3. The material is concise and clearly written.	Strongly agree			Strongly disagree	
	(1)	(2)	(3)	(4)	(5)
4. The material presented is . . .	Poor				Excellent
	(1)	(2)	(3)	(4)	(5)
5. To what degree will this material be usable in providing patient care?	Limited			Highly beneficial	
	(1)	(2)	(3)	(4)	(5)
6. The level of material presented is . . .	Too simple				Too advanced
	(1)	(2)	(3)	(4)	(5)
7. The overall quality of this handbook is . . .	Poor				Excellent
	(1)	(2)	(3)	(4)	(5)

Glossary

AIDS: Acquired immunodeficiency syndrome.

ARC: AIDS-related complex.

CD4: 62-kDa cell-surface glycoprotein on T-helper lymphocytes that is the specific virus receptor for HIV; HIV infection is associated with a loss of CD4 from infected T lymphocytes.

CD4 lymphocyte: Comprises approximately 60 percent of the T-lymphocyte population; contains effectors for delayed hypersensitivity and inducers for killer T-cell generation, B-cell differentiation into immunoglobulin-secreting plasma cells, and active suppressor-cell development.

CD8: Cell-surface glycoprotein on T-suppressor lymphocytes.

CD8 lymphocyte: Comprises approximately 30 percent of the lymphocyte population; contains effectors for killer T cells and other cells that suppress cell-mediated reactivities and immunoglobulin production.

CD4:CD8 ratio: Ratio of the number of CD4 lymphocytes to the number of CD8 lymphocytes; CD4 cells are depleted during HIV infection.

ELISA: Enzyme-linked immunosorbent assay; used to detect antibodies to multiple viral proteins.

HIV: Human immunodeficiency virus; member of the family Retroviridae (retroviruses), subfamily Lentivirinae (lentiviruses).

HIV antigens: translational protein products of the HIV gene (p = protein; gp = glycoprotein; the number is the molecular mass in kilodaltons:
p18, p24, gp41, gp120, gp160.

HIV genes:

Accessory (regulatory) genes:

nef: negative factor (previously known as 3'-*orf*).
rev: regulator of expression of virion proteins (previously know as *art/trs*).
tat: transactivator (previously known as *tat* III).
vif: virion infectivity factor (previously known as *sor*).
vpr: viral protein R.
vpu: viral protein U.

Structural genes (each codes for one or more proteins expressed in infected cells or in the mature virus:

gag: encodes the major core proteins.
pol: encodes two proteins with reverse transcriptase activity and the nuclease-integrase protein p31.
env: encodes a 160-kDa glycoprotein.

HTLV-I, -II: Human T-lymphotropic viruses.

IL-2: Interleukin-2; a glycoprotein lymphokine released by T lymphocytes when stimulated with an antigen.

Incidence: The number of new cases of a disease occurring over a period of time; a rate.

Lentiviruses: Subfamily of the family Retroviridae; cause slowly progressive diseases with lymphotropic and neurotropic features in humans and ungulates; HIV is the only known human lentivirus.

Oncoviruses: Viruses that cause many animal malignancies and characteristically immortalize cells in vitro.

PCP: *Pneumocytis carinii* pneumonia; opportunistic infection often seen in patients with AIDS.

PCR: Polymerase chain reaction; in vitro enzymatic technique used to amplify selected portions of a genome, thus allowing detection of HIV sequences.

Prevalence: The number of cases of a disease at a specific point in time.

Provirus: Double-stranded DNA intermediate in the replication cycle of retroviruses; often integrates into the host-cell genome, but may take an extrachromosomal, circular form.

Retrovirus: Virus characterized by a unique, viral-encoded enzyme called *reverse transcriptase*.

Reverse transcriptase: Retroviral enzyme that synthesizes DNA from RNA in a reverse flow of genetic transcription.

Seroconversion: Change in antibody status from negative to positive in response to a challenge to the immune system; demonstrated by serologic assay.

Western blot: Common confirmatory test used to detect antibodies to specific HIV viral proteins.

Zidovudine: 3'-azido-2'-3'-dideoxythymidine (formerly azidothymidine, AZT); the only anti-HIV agent approved by the U.S. Food and Drug Administration; inhibits HIV replication in vitro.

Index

Page references in *italic* indicate tables; page references in **boldface** indicate illustrations.